The Light Diet

How the Power of
Loving Yourself
Can Change Your Bodyshape
Forever!

Think light.
Feel light.
Be light.
Love your body.
Love your mind.
Love your emotions.
Love your spirit.

Become the true you
And set yourself free!

by Elisabeth Constantine

First published by Findhorn Press 2005

ISBN 1–84409–044-2

British Library Cataloguing-in-Publication Data.
A catalogue record for this book is available from
the British Library.

Edited by Lynn Barton
Cover by Thierry Bogliolo
Internal design by Karin Bogliolo
All photographs © Elisabeth Constantine 2005

Printed and bound by WS Bookwell, Finland

Published by
Findhorn Press
305a The Park, Findhorn
Forres IV36 3TE
Scotland, UK
tel 01309 690582
fax 01309 690036
e-mail: info@findhornpress.com

www.findhornpress.com

Contents

Dedication

This book is dedicated in memory and celebration
of the life of my soul sister Karen.
You live in our hearts forever!
To my family and all my friends
whom I love dearly.

All we need is love...

I would like to say thank you from my heart to God, the creator,
to my beloved Grandmaster and guide Sheikh Muhammad Nazim,
who has nourished my spirit, mind, body and soul
with the limitless power of his divine love
and to Sheikh Ahmad Dede for coming into my life
and enriching it in such a beautiful way.
A big thank you to my publishers, to Lynn my wonderful editor
and Carol and Sabine for their invaluable input.
I thank David Cousins, my former spiritual mentor, for his love and
understanding, which I appreciate deeply to this very day,
the angels and beings of light and my teachers in spirit,
especially Mavlana Jalaluddin Rumi, whose divine heartbeat reverberates
throughout the universes.
Thank you to all my wonderful friends for loving me the way you do.
You know who you are. I love you all!
A special thank you goes to my light sister Valerie
for her support with this project.
And last but ot least a very big thank you to my clients, healing students and
workshop participants for teaching me what I needed to learn.

...We are all One...

The Great Invocation

From the point of light within the mind of God
Let light stream forth into the minds of men.
Let light descend on earth.

From the point of love within the heart of God
Let love stream forth into the hearts of men.
May love return to earth.

From the centre where the will of God is known
Let purpose guide the little wills of men –
The purpose which the Masters know and serve.

From the centre which we call the race of men
Let the plan of love and light work out
And may it seal the door where evil dwells.

Let light and love and power restore the plan on earth.

Blessings to you all, dear readers,

In deepest gratitude I live.

In deepest gratitude I love.

In deepest gratitude I offer

what I have to give.

May the light of your own heart

illuminate your body, mind and soul.

May this light shine brightly

and illuminate the darkest corner of your being.

May love and light reign supreme in your life on earth.

I honour the light in each and every one of you!

With many blessings, your soul sister

and fellow traveller in the light,

Introduction: *The journey begins*

"A journey of a thousand miles must begin with a single step."
—Lao Tzu

To step fully into the light, we first must journey into the darkness of matter. To make the invisible visible, the light has to show up the dark. Once the shadows have been made visible, the light will transmute all darkness. The journey on which you are about to embark will take you through the layers of your past conditioning forever upwards towards the ultimate goal, the light of your own divine self. Thus utilising God's love, which IS the light, you will become the light. Loving yourself and all of creation equally, is the ultimate destination of your journey to the light. Then you will realise that in truth we are all ONE and that you have never been separated from God's love.

As with every journey, the one which lies ahead of you will have its ups and downs. All of us currently incarnated on this earth are on the same journey at this moment in time. Some will be aware of that fact, others not. In truth we are searching for the light, for our true identity, for our divine self, for God who is the "in-dweller".

Having been born with "spiritual amnesia", we have forgotten our divine origin, the nature of the true self, always present beneath the surface of the conditioned personality.

The content of this workbook is designed to guide you on your journey back to your true, divine nature, shining the light and love of God and the angels on your path along the way.

However, it is the love you will develop for yourself that is the key to the positive changes you will be able to make on your travels through the realms of your body, mind, emotions and spirit. To this end, this workbook will encourage you again and again to have trust and faith, and to "let go, let God". It will teach you the skills you need to accept yourself unconditionally the way you are right here, right now.

You may have heard of the concept of "tough love". Loving ourselves and others unconditionally is not a soft option; it is often tough love in action, as unconditional love equals truth and the sword of truth may induce pain when cutting through the layers of our conditioned feelings and behaviours.

"Truth, like surgery, may hurt, but it cures."
—Han Suyin

Such tough love can liberate us from the emotional and mental baggage we have been carting around with us. As our body, mind and emotions resist every change at every point and a little coaxing just does not do the job; for true change can only occur when

we make a real commitment,

As you travel to the core of your true self, you may encounter dark and painful emotions previously hidden from your conscious awareness. Allow yourself to go within, to feel these emotions and then release and let go of them; this workbook will give you the tools you need to do this safely.

(If you are working with particularly difficult, traumatic memories or events, please do not hesitate to ask for help from your fellow brothers and sisters who are experts in their field. Asking for help is synonymous with accepting love and is an important part of your healing. Consulting the help section at the end of this book will enable you to find the assistance that is right for you.)

I encourage you to stay with me on this journey and not to give up. It will all be worth it in the end! Remember to work at your own pace and to be kind and gentle to yourself along the way, giving yourself lots of treats as you move forward into the light of your divine self.

Your own soul is your greatest ally on the path to self-discovery and will speak to you through the language of your emotions. Listen carefully, even thought the feelings that arise may at times be unsettling, uncomfortable and even frightening. Know that you are never alone, that God and the angels are always watching over you and that you are deeply loved at all times, even though you may not be aware of it at present.

> *"The time has come to turn your heart into a temple of fire.*
> *Your essence is gold hidden in dust.*
> *To reveal its splendour you need to burn in the fire of love."*
> *—Rumi*

Step-by-step, as you develop more and more love for yourself, you will be getting more and more into "divine shape".

First your negative thoughts will drop from you, then your negative emotions will fall away and, last but not least, your body will adjust itself to its divine natural weight. Your success is divinely assured. The true you will emerge, perfect, in the image God has intended for you.

A note on language

Throughout the workbook the terms "God", "source" and "universe" have been used interchangeably for the divine, as have the pronouns "He" and "She".

Part 1:
How we ended up with our present body-shape

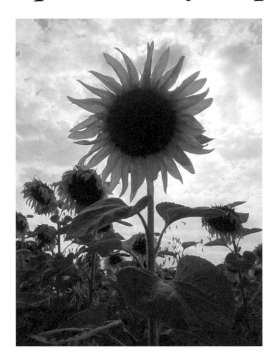

"The unexamined life is not worth living."
— *Plato*

The conditioned self

How did I get to this place, you might ask yourself. How, on earth, did I arrive here, with this imperfect life, this less than perfect body, my spirit dampened by the hardships I have endured?

You have arrived at this moment in time, just like a freight train, after a long journey, huffing and puffing under the weight of pulling its many wagons.

This weight that you have been carrying with you throughout your life consists of old, unresolved issues, suppressed emotions and negative mental patterns formed over many lifetimes. This baggage is what has been slowing you down, hampering your progress and often stopping you from creating and enjoying the life and the body shape you deserve.

How did you allow this to happen? Most of us have fallen victim to the conditioning of our childhood and teenage years. About 70% of your personality may have been projected on to you by your nearest and dearest, and by society at large. The person you see in the mirror is you by name, but not the true you. The feelings you feel and the thoughts you think do not belong to you in the sense that they do not truly originate from a neutral you. The influence of the emotional, social, religious and political environment you grew up in has fashioned you into the person you see in the mirror.

It's interesting to note that the word 'personality' comes from the Greek word 'persona', meaning mask. This is the mask of protection from potentially harmful outside influences, which we learn very quickly, even as a small children, to put on. This is the same smiling mask you now wear, so that everybody loves you.

As children our parents or carers are our whole world. We might not have got on with them, yet we still copied their behaviour, their way of life and much more.

Many of us were moulded and fashioned like a piece of clay into the child our parents wanted to see, or often, into the child they themselves wanted to be when they were young. So off you went to ballet class, although you hated it and really wanted to do sports. Or perhaps you were made to do horse riding, when in truth you were terribly afraid, but even more ashamed to say so. Some of our parents also tell us how much they've sacrificed to bring us up and give us things. Thus with these feelings of guilt foisted onto us we now feel less than free to be ourselves. So is it any wonder that we don't even dare to talk about our dreams, let alone attempt to make them into a reality for ourselves?

Moreover, guilt is a prime source of the disturbed behaviour patterns that lead to the development of eating disorders on the physical level, and of depression and anxiety on the emotional or mental levels.

The materialistic values of society, particularly in the western world, have affected most of us as well. Self-worth is thought to reside in becoming rich, powerful and famous.

The true values of love for one another and of living a life in service to humanity, not in a dreary, suppressed way, but in a fun way, with a job and/or way of life that is loved and enjoyed, have been almost lost and forgotten; that someone who sits on the beach all day thinking loving thoughts and minding their own business is just as worthwhile a human being as someone who sits in an office playing the stock exchange is inconceivable to many.

So, if you were not a child who happily and easily conformed to your parents' wishes and societies dictates, it is likely that your childhood and especially your teenage years were difficult at best.

If you were a child who only pretended to go along suppressing your true feelings, letting them boil and fester away inside, you may have grown up into an angry, disillusioned adult, never quite knowing why you turned out that way. These unresolved emotions can be carried into your adult life and unconsciously projected on to other people and situations, turning many a positive possibility into a negative outcome.

To somehow function in these difficult circumstances, you may have developed certain coping mechanisms, for example eating or not eating, so that you could feel in control of your life.

Conditioning can be obvious and fairly easy to spot, but it can also be extremely subtle, having enmeshed the child in an invisible web of projections.

Now as an adult, you may not even know yourself, may not know how to divide the true self from the false, projected self.

Showing you how to do this is one of the objectives of this book.

"By three methods we may learn wisdom.
First by reflection, which is noblest;
second by imitation, which is the easiest;
and third by experience, which is the bitterest."
—Confucius

Pregnancy and birth trauma

As the latest research shows, we may already have been affected by the behaviour of our parents and by outside influences while still a tiny embryo in the womb.

Not only does the embryo suffer from the mother's smoking, drinking, bad diet, poor sleeping habits, etc., it is also influenced by any emotional, mental and physical trauma the mother, and to a lesser extent, the father, goes through.

Researchers have discovered that babies in the womb can recognise the voices of their parents and other nearest and dearest. So, if your mother was in an abusive relationship, mentally, physically or emotionally, while being pregnant with you, you would have experienced this negative energy and it will have stayed with you into your adult life.

Negative pre-birth experiences may show up later as irrational fears or resentments towards the abuser or others who remind you of the abuser, thus influencing your behaviour patterns and the way you relate to the people close to you. It can certainly lead to issues around trust and intimacy.

One of the biggest events in our lives is our birth itself. If your birth was swift and smooth, without any traumatic incidences, you are one of the lucky ones, rejoice.

Unfortunately many more of us have not been so lucky, having gone through considerable birth trauma.

Research, particularly through the processes of hypnotic regression and re-birthing, has shown that birth trauma can give rise to all manner of emotional, mental and physical problems. With many of my clients I have observed deep-seated fears, the root of which turned out to be a traumatic, often prolonged, sometimes also violent birth.

The events of our birth are perfectly preserved in our consciousness. Perhaps you had the umbilical cord around your neck and were nearly choked by it, feeling you might die at any minute. If so, in later life, you may suffer a fear of suffocation by harmless things, like a tight polo neck jumper or the zipper on a cardigan. It might even lead to a far greater fear of death, or of being killed in some unknown circumstances.

Fear is often the constant companion of the child who has endured birth trauma. Unaware where this fear is coming from, we may seek to protect ourselves from any more harm by over-eating, so that the layers of fat form a barrier between us and the hostile outside world. At the same time we may also put emotional and mental barriers in place, which will block any incoming energy, including the energy of love. In such cases our emotional and mental wires having been crossed by the trauma we have endured. Love becomes equated with pain and we may fear that being loved would somehow hurt us and even cause our death and demise.

Often what we fear the most is exactly what deep inside we long for, thus leading us into a vicious cycle of attracting love, then immediately rejecting it, so as to avoid hurt. A deep resentment at having been born and for living a life that is not fulfilling often follows.

To disengage from this cycle of destruction, if you have suffered a traumatic birth, or suspect you might have, please see a therapist, such as a qualified hypnotherapist or rebirther, to release the trauma once and for all. Both approaches have been extremely successful in healing such events.

"Nothing in life is to be feared.
It is only to be understood."
—Marie Curie

Childhood abuse

Currently there are many victims of sexual abuse who are waking up from the slumber of these suppressed painful events and speaking out about their terrible ordeals.

Thank God, we as a society are now ready to listen to them and support them to the best of our abilities, and many government and private initiatives have been put into place to further the healing of those terrible wounds.

Abuse, whether in childhood, teenage or early adult years, is much more common than I had ever anticipated. In my private practice over a fifteen-year period, I found an astonishing 40% of my clients had suffered abuse, of a sexual nature mainly by their parents, carers or other close family or friends.

To compensate for the lack of love, the shame, guilt, anger, resentment and the host of other emotions they experienced, these clients often use food, alcohol or drugs as a way of coping with, or dulling, the emotional, mental and sometimes physical pain. Often this leads to a variety of long-term addictive behaviours.

With many of these clients I noticed a change in body-shape after some time in therapy. Most overweight clients would report a loss of body fat over a period of time, and people who had previously not been able to gain weight were suddenly able to do so.

It became clear to me that these clients had in a variety of ways used food to replace love. In the case of overeating or binge eating, they had been substituting food for the love that had been lacking in their lives and which they craved for so much. In the case of undereating, they felt unworthy of love and unable to receive it and therefore punished themselves by withholding food from their bodies, although for reasons of which they were not consciously aware.

The environment we live in

Even though it is ultimately the mind that creates our reality, where and how we live and the choices we make regarding our general well being, will have a substantial effect on our mental, emotional, physical and spiritual health. Living in a city puts strains on our physical and maybe also on our mental health, as city life is normally far more stressful than living in a nice cottage in the countryside. Whether we live in the city or the countryside, fresh air and exercise are of vital importance for a healthy way of life as is the quality and duration of your sleep.

The foods we choose to eat will affect us greatly; you are what you eat, remember. Eating organically grown and GM-free food, abstaining from consuming flesh (unless the animal has been slaughtered the kosher or halal way) and sticking to a vegetarian diet will affect our health in a positive manner. What we are absorbing into our body is the energy of the food, and the vibratory pattern of the food will affect our own vibratory pattern. If the food we eat is of a lower energy rate than we are, it will literally bring us down.

This is why, after eating certain foods, we might not only feel physically unwell, but also even feel depressed or full of emotions for which we have no logical explanation. Food intolerance accounts for a whole host of symptoms, such as bloating, and general tiredness after food intake. I would suggest that if you have such symptoms, you see a professional kinesiologist to uncover what you're allergic to, so that the problem can be eliminated. If you tend to eat fast or pre-prepared food, be mindful of blessing it, as food, like any other substance, will absorb the energy of the person who has been handling it. If someone was angry or upset at the time of preparing the food, all of those bad vibrations will have been absorbed into it.

After you have eaten this dish, you will most likely have some form of upset or discomfort, depending on how sensitive you are. (It could be the sensation of a stone landing in your stomach accompanied by a feeling of being unsettled.)

What prevents us from being the perfect body-shape?

Beneath the many, papery layers of onion skin, lies the pristine, glistening white onion. Beneath the layers of false conditioning lies the true self, which is already perfect at its core. Thus the layers of the false personality, the persona, the mask, need to be finally peeled away to reveal a being of light and love.

For this process to take place, many changes have to occur. We may have to change our way of thinking and reassess our emotional processes. We may have to change how we interact with others and how we act and react in certain situations or circumstances. And finally we may have to change our diet and lifestyle.

The hitch is that we all resist change. "Better the devil I know, than the one I don't," is our general modus operandi.

Change is indeed a frightening process. Every conditioned fibre in our being, on all the levels of existence, the mind, the emotions and the body, resists it. The goal posts are being moved. Will we be able to keep up with the progress? Do we have it in us to adjust to new, unknown situations or inner states of being?

To effect lasting change in our lives we will each of us have to find out what truly makes our soul sing.

If our heart is not in it, as in so many diets or lifestyle changes, we may have previously attempted, nothing will change for the better – or if it does then it can only be maintained for a short period of time, leading eventually to more frustration and anger at ourselves.

What has prevented us from being not only the perfect body-shape, but also from being in perfect mental, emotional and spiritual shape has been a resistance to love; a resistance to the love God has been, and still is, trying to lavish upon us – and, crucially, a resistance to our own self-love.

At the heart of the matter, what is needed is true love for the self, love without conditions attached to it, love that means total positive self-regard and self-acceptance for who and what we are at this moment in time. This is how God loves us and always will love us free of judgement, free of criticism, free of any prejudices about who we are and what we have or haven't done in this or any other lifetime. This love is the best tool, the best weapon, to cut away, dissolve, release and let go of all old attachments and addictions so that we are free to become our true selves co-creators with God on this lovely planet, called mother earth.

This love is the foremost ingredient in the light diet.

The only thing which will make your soul sing jubilantly is the sweet melody of unconditional love and light!

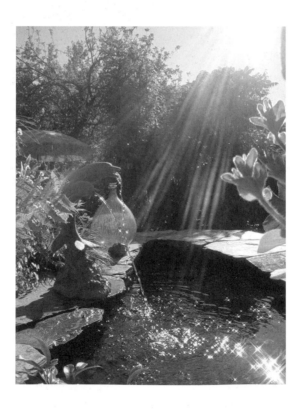

Part 2:
God matters

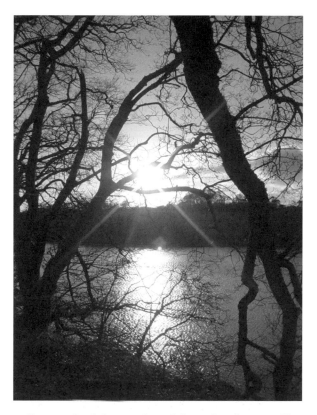

"I searched for God and found only myself.
I searched for myself and found only God."
—Sufi proverb

Who are we?

How we feel shapes what we think about ourselves. In your heart of hearts, do you feel good about yourself? Most of us do not.

We may feel ourselves to be failures, having not been able to live up to the – unrealistic, inappropriate – expectations of our family, peer group or society at large. We may even feel that we are sinners, having acted in ways which were not compatible with our social conditioning, but which felt totally natural and comfortable to us.

Sounds familiar?

Were you told by your family not to have expectations beyond your social, cultural and personal standing?

Were you accused of daydreaming, of wasting time in idle fantasy or useless pursuits?

And were you told, often repeatedly, that you just would not be good enough to achieve such a dream or goal?

If the answer to even only one of these questions is yes, then your life-force, the totality of your soul energy, will have been stifled from an early age onwards, leading to parts of yourself, the creative parts, literally excusing themselves and returning back to your higher spirit self, where they still dwell waiting from an invitation from your lower self, which is housed in your physical body, to join you and become active in your mission as co-creator with God in this lifetime.

So, all in all you may see yourself as a miserable human being, a mortal, in a physical shell – a body – which is getting older and more useless as you watch, with an unruly mind which is constantly trying to dominate you and with emotions, which at times, run away with you and threaten to overwhelm you.

A bleak outlook for the future ensues from such a limited view of ourselves. No wonder, that in order to compensate for this sorry state of affairs, we reach for food, drink, drugs or other substances and activities to comfort ourselves with.

In fact, the exact opposite of who we think we are is the truth.

You are a being of light having a human experience, not a human being having an experience of light!

Our true essence is the soul, which dwells in the chamber of the heart, in the physical body, until we draw our last breath, when it returns back to source, to our divine higher spirit self.

There it rests until it is ready to incarnate into another body, to begin a new life on earth, until it finally knows itself to be God – to be the light – and it does not have to journey anymore, forever dwelling in divine bliss.

The fabric of the soul is woven from God's unconditional love, which is manifested as light. The soul is indestructible, a divine spark of God's energy, its light-quotient, hopefully, increasing from lifetime to lifetime.

The body, the emotions and the mind are the tools, which the soul has chosen, in order to learn about itself and to finally experience itself as God.

As with all tools, we have to learn how to use them. However in a society that is mainly orientated towards outward, materialistic values, the inner workings of the mind and the emotions have been largely ignored, being deemed unimportant; so we are not really taught how to use our mind and emotions efficiently.

Spiritual education on this planet is mainly connected to religious teachings, often very much enmeshed in dogma and structure, which hardly allows a joyful, self-empowered spirituality to develop. The awesome truth that the individual actually is "God in action", is a dangerous threat to most religious organisations and those who lead them.

> *"My religion is to live and die without regret."*
> *—Milarepa*

God is not, as we have been told, a being apart from us.

God is the "in-dweller" he resides within our very being and we reside within Him.

We and God are intrinsically linked; we are made of God-fabric – and so is the whole of creation. All is interpenetrated, interwoven with the light and the love of God, with the light and the love of our higher divine self.

We can neither divide God from us, nor can we add God to us; God is part of us, and has been forever, never changing, always present.

Wherever we look, we are looking at God, in one form, expression or another.

Living contemplation: the nature of God

When you get up tomorrow morning, decide to "look for God" in all that you see and experience.

To successfully complete this living contemplation, you need to make a special effort to open your heart and mind, enabling you to discover the "God within", which is often hidden from sight.

Turn your attention to finding the divine expression in everyone and everything, look for it in the people you live and work with, in the tree, shrub or little birds you encounter on your way to work or while walking the baby in the park.

You may find God in a passing glance or the smile of a complete stranger…

Look for signs of light, love and joy that can be found in all creation. Watch and search carefully, as beauty is often veiled in the seemingly ugly and it is the nature of the conditioned self not to look beyond appearances.

You will be surprised by what you have found by the end of your day.

You will have encountered love, light and joy, sure signs of the presence of God in places you never dreamt of.

❀   ❀   ❀

"If you seek the kernel, then you must break the shell.
And likewise, if you would know the reality of nature,
you must destroy the appearance, and the further you go beyond
the appearance the nearer you will see the essence."
—Meister Eckhart

Love, the universal superglue

The invisible essence, the love of God, which is manifested as light, is "the universal superglue" which holds this universe together. We are each part of this magical universe, being a vital, irreplaceable piece of a giant cosmic jigsaw puzzle. Without our participation the divine plan – namely, the illumination through God's love and light, the enlightenment of the whole planet earth, and the birthing of mother earth into a star, – is not able to unfold. It cannot be completed, if each of us does not take our seat at the throne of God as a co-creator with God.

The more love, the more divine superglue we have in our hearts and are willing to freely give, the more peace and harmony will be spread throughout all of God's creation.

You have the power. You are a co-creator with God.

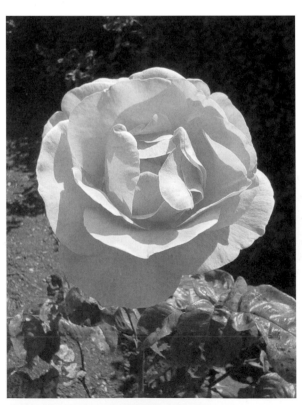

"And when you work with love you bind yourself to yourself,
and to one another, and to God."
—Kahlil Gibran, The Prophet

This is why our aim must be first to know ourselves, then to fill ourselves with love; we must strive continuously to become a vessel for love, and finally the vessel itself, the ego will dissolve and we will become love.

A love which is pure, knowing no bounds, a love nothing can stop, a love nothing can distort, a love nothing can manipulate or change in any way.

God is part of us and we are part of God, therefore the whole of creation is part of you, all your soul brothers and sisters, the plants, the animals, the rocks and the stars and planets in the sky.

"The self is a circle whose centre is everywhere
and whose circumference is nowhere."
—C. G. Jung

Letter to God

Please set aside at least half an hour of undisturbed time for this written exercise. Take paper and pen and allow yourself to relax by taking several deep breaths. Breathe in love and light on the in-breath and release and let go on the out-breath. Contemplate the notion that you are a co-creator with God. This will inevitably bring up a whole host of questions.

When you are ready begin to write your letter to God.

Start by writing, "Dear God my name is .... and I would like you answer the following questions. I thank you in advance for giving me all the answers I need." Add your signature.

Now having established communication with God, take a nice, deep breath, breathing in love and light, and when you are ready begin to write down a question and quickly jot down the answer that will come floating into your mind.

Do not hesitate to write what will, at the beginning, feel like your own thoughts; trust that they are not, as they truly come from God. Continue to write down all your questions and God's answers in this way. When you have finished, give thanks.

You will find that the words you have written in answer to your questions will have a different quality than your own words would have had. God's wisdom and love will shine from the page.

Trust the insights contained within and repeat this exercise as often as you like.

The more frequently you practise it, the easier it will become.

The here and now factor

"We choose our joys and sorrows long before we experience them."
—*Kahlil Gibran, The Prophet*

What each of us thinks, feels and does will have an effect on the whole and what the rest of humanity thinks, feels and does affects each of us.

To know and accept this truth brings with it both great responsibilities and great opportunities.

An important premise of this book, which we will discuss in more detail later, is that we each create our own reality. If we accept this premise with our current thinking and conditioned programming still intact and active, we will very quickly feel totally overwhelmed and depressed by it.

There is only one remedy to this malady. We must make the decision, right here, right now – as the now is all there is – that the past is in the past and your future just a fantasy, a projection, an expectation of sorts. We must grab hold of the power that being in the now affords us, by being fully present and letting go of the past in its entirety, with all that it has meant to us physically, emotionally, mentally. We must let go of any old spiritual oaths and beliefs as well and release also all our expectations about the future.

Practising the following affirmation will help you to separate from the past and release your expectations of the future, propelling you into the here and now and thus releasing yourself from attachments to the past and future affirmation.

Ask for help from the healing angels and the beings of light stating out loud 3 times:

I AM THE I AM!

I now release all attachments, be they of a physical, emotional, mental or spiritual nature that do not serve my highest good and the highest good of all creation.

I release all attachments from my conscious and subconscious mind, through all times and all dimensions, into the light, to be transmuted by the light.

And so be it.

And so be it.

And so be it.

❀ ❀ ❀

Give thanks for the support you have received and repeat daily for as long as it seems appropriate and until you feel a shift in energy, which will manifest itself as a feeling of being lighter and much happier to move forward in life.

We are each responsible for our lives, the thoughts we think, the words we speak, the things we do, the choices we make. Contrary to what society says, we are allowed to make mistakes and, very importantly, we are allowed to backtrack and change our minds as often as we like; nothing is set in stone. We are responsible for ourselves and other people are in turn responsible for their own actions. (Naturally we care for our children and loved ones and treat our soul brothers and sisters and mother earth with the same love, respect and kindness we would like to be treated with.)

As you practise the affirmation, you will start to feel a sense of freedom in your heart. You will feel that the burdens of the past have actually dropped away and the high and sometimes very specific expectations for the future you had of yourself and others will no longer give you sleepless nights. You will start to get a measure of true freedom, the freedom you need to live a life fully in the now, making good choices and decisions in the now that will shape your future. You no longer waste your life-force in lamenting the past or in projecting your valuable energy into a future scenario which might never happen.

By being in the here and now, you will simply have so much more energy to function, available to you. Now you know, why the present is indeed a "present" a truly magical gift, which God is offering you.

Your mind will resist this change, trying to pull you back into the past or forward into the future in order not to have to deal with your present reality. Please be gentle with yourself while engaging in the "coming into the now" process, as it will take time.

"What lies behind us and what lies before us are tiny matters, compared to what lies within us."
—Ralph Waldo Emerson

Soul communication

The soul, seated in the chamber of the heart, speaks to us through our feelings. I am sure that it is true for you too that no matter how much you think something might be good for you, if it does not feel right, you most likely won't do it. And if you override your feelings then nine out of ten times it won't work out!

Why are the promptings of the soul superior to the workings of the mind?

Because the soul receives information from our higher divine God-self, which in turn is connected to the source of all there is, the source of love and light, namely, God.

A silver cord – which acts like a high-speed link and is visible to clairvoyants – connects the soul directly to our higher divine God–self. The power connecting the soul with the higher self is the power of the intuition. This is an energy that is far superior to the fabrications of the mind and the thought processes, which are mainly conditioned.

The intellect on the other hand – the power of reason – is the faculty, which, when properly developed, allows us to discern between one thought form and another; this ability differentiates the human mind from the instinctive nature of the animal mind. If we look into how great innovations have happened, we find that there was always a quantum leap involved. All great innovators and explorers of the frontiers of science have been great visionaries; Einstein could have come up with his Quantum Theory only by applying his intuitive faculties and a good dose of trust and faith in his own vision.

If we listen to our intuition we are allowing the soul to speak to our higher, divine all-knowing God-self.

This God-self, which is a spark of the divine, will in turn deliver the information we want via the intuition, bypassing the conditioned mind.

This is in fact direct communication with God, who is identical with your higher, divine self!

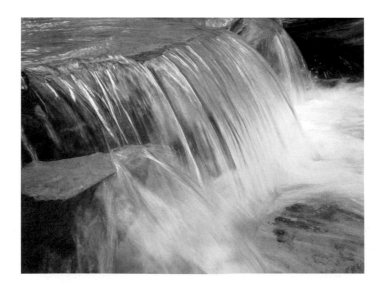

"Your vision will become clear only when you look into your heart...
Who looks outside, dreams.
Who looks inside, awakens."
—C. G. Jung

Living Contemplation:
Conversations with your soul

Make time to visit your favourite outdoor place, be it a park, woodland or a beach.

Choose a spot where you can be undisturbed for some time.

Sit comfortably, take a few deep breaths and close your eyes.

Now, physically, put your left hand on your heart and your right hand over it.

You are now connecting with your soul.

What does it feel like to touch your soul?

You may find a warm, soft, comforting feeling flowing through your whole body.

Now, in your mind, begin to talk to your soul.

Say "Hello my dearest soul" and say thank you for the journey it has undertaken on your behalf.

Express your gratitude for the hardships it has been through for the benefit of your learning.

As you do so you will experience feelings of joy flooding your very being; this is your soul responding to your gratitude and love for it.

When you are ready, ask your soul if it would like to communicate anything particular to you at this moment in time.

You may get a strong emotion or a specific thought coming to you; just relax and let it happen.

Alternatively you may not feel anything special at all.

Do not force the issue; your soul may want to communicate something specific on another occasion.

In your own good time, say thank you and promise your soul that you will make these conversations a regular practice.

Take your hands off your heart and have a little stretch before you get up.

You will find the world to be a brighter place after a conversation with your soul.

Enjoy!

Part 3:
Light matters

"The clear light at the centre changes everything."
—Rumi

We are light and love

God=Light, this is the light of God which has created us and the whole of creation at large.

Light=love, this is the creative energy of light which exists and expands through the all-powerful force of unconditional love.

We are completely composed of light on the "outside" and on the "inside".

Our bodies are made up of matter, and matter is made up of light. Matter vibrates at a low frequency. (It could be called "frozen light", as matter – and the body – to all intents and purposes seem to be solid.) Thus we are composed of light on the outside and light is also ensconced within us in the diamond of our heart, the soul. Every fibre of our being is thus "light-filled".

The power of love, the light of God, vibrates within us and within all animate and inanimate objects. The higher the light = love – quotient contained in the person, animal, plant, rock or fabricated object, the higher its frequency will be.

A happy, joyful, loving person will vibrate at the highest light-rate, a miserable, frightened, hateful one at the lowest.

The heart is the primary distributor of physical energy for the body; for it is the seat of the soul, and it is the soul that stores and distributes light and love within our being. Light=love is the spiritual super-food not only for us but for all of creation.

It is an energy vibration on a high frequency which causes us to not only feel good, but to extend our energies outward, and through this process we begin to create easily and joyfully.

Our aim, therefore, must be, first and foremost, to bring as much light and love into our whole lives as possible; be it through our thoughts, our emotions, our bodies, our diet and the activities we perform. The more we respect ourselves for who we truly are, a spark of the divine, the more we will reject all which is "not love". How do we know what is not true love?

The soul will speak to us through the language of feeling. We can trust our feelings and use our "in-tuition" to confirm them. Life, if we have trust and faith, will teach us all we need to know. God and the universe are on our side!

Once our whole being, body, mind and emotions are truly anchored in love, we will uplift anybody and anything around us that vibrates at a lower frequency. People who are depressed and sad will lighten up, when we give them a smile from the heart. We have all met people who are referred to as "a ray of sunshine" by their friends and acquaintances. These are our soul brothers and soul sisters who allow rays of love to shine freely into the world from the centre of their hearts, their souls and thus uplift all those around them into a higher vibration. Not only can our light=love quotient be increased but so can that of our pets and other animals, as can that of physical places where we work and dwell, as well as that of objects, products and ventures.

When the craftsperson builds a cabinet with skill and love, its light=love quotient is high, far higher than one produced in a factory. There is more light and love in any product, be it a pizza or a pair of shoes, that is created with passion and commitment than in one that is produced solely to make a profit, and a business that is run with love is always sure to succeed.

> *"Love nurtures all things that grow;*
> *it harmonises and unites."*
> *—Paramahansa Yogananda*

There are other ways, of course, to increase our light=love quotient. It is possible to use our sacred breath, historically seen as the basic constituent and source of all life. In the ancient Hindu tradition, the sacred breath was prana, in the ancient Chinese it was chi and in the Kabbalah, the Jewish mystical tradition, it was the astral light.

Indian yogis, "the light eaters" have been known to survive solely on light for decades and in the west, the Breatharians believe we can live on light and air. As light=love=God, this might indeed be possible. However, there are some crucial factors to consider. The most important one is that eating is closely related to our emotional needs. The needier we are, the more we eat. When we go through periods of loneliness or stress, many of us reach for food or drink for comfort. It would be possible to live on light and air only if we had cleared all our unresolved emotions, but how many of us have done that?

We can, however, increase our light=love quotient through our sacred breath by practising breathing exercises, several of which are given in detail later in this book.

The power of blessing

I cannot stress enough the value of the act of blessing as a way of raising the light=love quotient in our food – and in every person and situation we meet. (The role of blessing in the process of forgiveness is explored in Part 5 The divine seal of blessing.)

The blessing of food is of the utmost importance. As all matter vibrates at various levels and we have ascertained that the more light=love is inherent in matter, the higher its vibration is, we can safely conclude that we would want to imbue our food with as much light=love as we possibly can.

From the point of light, the real function of the digestive system is the condensation of spiritual energy, as the more light you absorb into your physical, mental and emotional body, the more your well-being increases, the longer you will live a happy, joyful, healthy and fulfilled life.

All foodstuff, be it liquids or solids, is also "frozen light", some of it "deep-frozen", with very little energy, and some just "chilled", with a lot more light-force left in it.

In order for us to be the body-shape we would love to be, we have to love ourselves accordingly. This means that the foodstuff we take in should at least match the love and care we have for ourselves. When all that "is not love" has been eliminated from our systems and when at the same time we only put "light substances" into our mouths, we will have, by the universal law of like attracts like, achieved our perfect body shape.

What is equally true, and just another way to look at this, is that at our core we are already perfect, all that needs to happen is for us to release our mental and emotional blockages, which will lead our physical weight to be balanced automatically.

Hence we must make sure that the substances we take into our systems are as pure, as light, as possible, so that we assimilate them without having to drop our vibratory rate to a lower level, which would, of course, be counterproductive.

The way to raise our energy-intake – besides carefully choosing fresh, possibly organically grown, GM-free, produce – is through blessing it.

As we bless something (somebody or a situation), we instantly raise its vibration.

The act of blessing – God's love and light streaming forth from the heart – fills the substance with light and transmutes any negativity inherent within it and so also acts as a great cleansing and disinfecting agency.

Since I started blessing my food regularly, I have never had any stomach upsets of any kind while travelling in countries like India, (famous for the Delhi-belly syndrome, which I have had the bad fortune to suffer from on numerous occasions prior to my blessing my food). The proof does always lie in the pudding, to me this is real, tangible physical proof that blessing works.

Blessing is a tool for magical transformation of murky matter of all sorts into light matter. A blessing can even be physically measured and documented by electro-photography, or Kirlian photography (named after Russian researcher Semyon Kirlian) which measures the aura, the electromagnetic field, around a person or object. When a healer attunes himself via contemplation or meditation, the energy field around him can be seen to grow in size. The same is true for the electromagnetic field around a loaf of bread when the housewife bakes and then blesses it. I remember as a child, my mother would draw three symbolic crosses with a knife on the top of the loaf, in order to bless it. The cooking of a cabbage in the microwave has the opposite effect, resulting in the living aura of the cabbage being almost completely destroyed. There is hardly any light=love=life-force energy, which is what truly feeds and sustains us, left, a fact which the manufacturers of microwave ovens are very aware of, hence the warning not to warm milk or baby food for infants! (The manufacturers surely know the effect the radiation has on food, why otherwise the warning for babies?) May this serve as a warning: if we microwave our food, the energy of the food will be almost completely lost; all there is left is fibre, ballast! The result: you need to eat more and more to feel full and satisfied.

Therefore, bless, bless, bless! Let us bless every bit of food we put into our mouths, every sip we drink and every lotion and potion we either ingest or rub onto our body. (Remembering that all substances rubbed onto the body get absorbed into the bloodstream via your largest organ, the skin, so beware especially of carcinogenic hair-dyes and hygiene products for women.) Moreover, the act of blessing empowers us. We are being consciously active, we are doing something for ourselves, we are loving ourselves by making sure that our foodstuff, and anything else we come in contact with, is of the highest possible light-rate. We are taking an important step towards being co-creators with God by actively increasing our light=love quotient, as loving ourselves unconditionally is what mother/father God truly wants for us.

Please consider using one of the following blessings. Once practised, they will take only seconds, but will increase the light=love quotient of your food tremendously.

BLESSING WITH GOLDEN LIGHT

Golden light is the universal healing light and intuitively you will choose the gold vibration to bless most of your food.

In your mind thank God and mother earth for the food you are about to bless.

Place both hands, palms facing down over your food.

Then visualise a beam of golden light above your head. Ask for the food to be blessed.

See the beam of golden light entering the top of your head, from there it flows via your third eye chakra, your throat chakra into your heart centre, into your lungs and from there down your arms into the palms of your hands, your palm chakras.

Finally the light flows into your food.

You will have an inner knowing when the process is done.

In general the more light the food contains, the less time is needed to bless it.

Give thanks .

BLESSING WITH SILVER LIGHT

Silver light has antiseptic properties, which is a very useful quality if you are faced with food you are not sure about.

This is a very valuable blessing when consuming food in foreign countries and also if you are aware that whoever cooked your food was in a bad mood or ill.

Please use exactly the same procedure, just visualise the beam of light to be silver.

The power of prayer

Amost potent tool for creating the reality of love and light in our lives is prayer. The most successful way to pray is not to just want something with our minds, but to feel intensely what we are praying for, to feel it with passion in our very hearts.

"Prayer is the best armour we have,
it is the key which opens the heart of God."
— Padre Pio

A prayer springing forth from a sincere heart devoted to light and love will always be answered in time, although it may take a little while. God-time, or divine timing, is not always human-time, hence the prayer "God please grant me patience". Our prayers, however, are always heard. They will be answered according to the divine plan, in divine timing, for the highest good of ourselves and of all sentient beings on this planet and of creation at large. When the window in time is right, the answer to our prayers will come. It may be through a feeling or an inspiration we have or through a messenger of God, one of our fellow soul brothers and sisters, or our guardian angel or guide may impress an answer. It may be through something we witness on television, watch in a movie or read in a book or newspaper.

Nature might even bring the answer to our prayers. A butterfly, representing spirit, might fly past the window at the precise moment we look out or we might hear the screeching of a wise owl at night, and infer that there is wisdom in waiting and being patient. A sudden gust of wind might blow on our daily walk, heralding the winds of change, or soft rain might fall, showing us that a release has taken place. If we are alert and watch for the answer in everything, in everybody and in all situations we will find it. If we make a supreme effort to learn to read the signs the universe is presenting to us, we will comprehend. If we have missed a sign or misunderstood it, in time it will come round again, until you have got the message.

At first the signs designed to catch our attention will be gentle. If we do not look or listen and pay attention or if we purposefully ignore the signs God is providing for us, then they get a little more emphatic. Often banging our heads or taking a fall or tumble is a sign for us to look out and, most of all, to look within to find out what is going on. Nothing happens at random; the seeming chaos we are surrounded with is actually in perfect divine order.

"God grant me the serenity to accept the things I cannot change;
courage to change the things I can;
and wisdom to know the difference."
—from the Serenity prayer

Prayer does, however, not mean that we hand over our lives to an outside force.

If we ask, "God, what do you want me to do?", the answer will be "Whatever you would most like to do, my child!" God has given us free will. This is a cosmic law, which cannot be overridden, not even by God. The universe, God, will support us in whatever we wish, if it is in accordance with divine will and divine law.

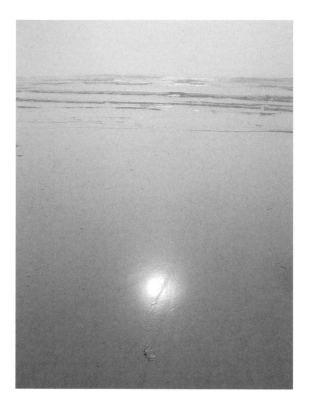

"Prayer is not asking.
It is a longing of the soul."
— Mahatma Gandhi

We are the creators of our own destiny

This brings us to another true saying, which is very much to the point. "Be careful what you wish for". What will make us truly happy cannot be found on the outside. Fame, fortune and possessions are just fleeting pleasures, subject to change. One minute we have them; the next minute they have evaporated into thin air. After all, there is nothing we can truly posses, except our own pure hearts filled with love, as we are truly only guardians of all material things.

If we strive to fill our hearts with happy, uplifting, joyful thoughts, they will serve as magnets drawing more joy, light and love to us. Needless to say, if our hearts are permanently filled with sorrow, grief and bitterness, we will also draw more of the same to ourselves. We cannot afford to stay in such a dark space for long; it may become a habit and what good is it doing anyone? Even in the worst scenario there is light at the end of the tunnel. The secret is to look intently for the light, as it is always there.

The reality we inhabit, that is, the physical plane in which we exist, functions through the duality, the positive and the negative; these produce light and dark, sweet and sour, hard and soft, male and female, yin and yang, and the cosmic law of cause and effect, the law of karma that governs the workings on planet earth. One aspect of the duality cannot exist without the other.

Life and death are two sides of the manifested eternal consciousness; the eternal pair of opposites, continuously inter-playing with each other, creates the diversity of life on planet earth.

This is why everything, be it termed good or evil, is part of the ONE divine creative energy, which the Zen Buddhists call Tao, the neutral creative energy, within which lies the potential to create what we humans on this planet want to create. So it's up to us to listen to our hearts and create heaven on earth and live in it happily forever after…

The law of free will gives each of us the choice of using God's energy for better or for worse. The power is in our hands.

The perfect divine plan allows us to consciously experience true unconditional love by letting us first experience what its opposite, namely conditional love, feels like. How much would we truly appreciate what we have in terms of health, wealth and knowledge, if we had not experienced, in this or any of our previous lives being poor, ill and uneducated? We would not truly value any of it, nor would we have sincere compassion for our soul brothers and soul sisters who are suffering at the moment. We couldn't relate to any suffering, even if we tried, as there would be no point of reference for us. We could only imagine how bad or good someone feels, but we would never truly know what's really going on inside their hearts, minds and bodies.

> *"There are as many nights as days,*
> *and the one is just as long as the other in the year's course.*
> *Even a happy life cannot be without a measure of darkness, and the word 'happy'*
> *would loose its meaning if it were not balanced by sadness."*
> —C. G. Jung

God's ultimate plan is for us to awaken from the illusion of matter, to realise who we are, sparks of the divine with all the same attributes that are inherent within mother/father God. For this purpose God has granted us the gift of the emotions, a wonderful gift, the most important teaching device, allowing the soul incarnated in the physical body to express its wisdom to us. A life devoid of emotions, solely lived in the mind, would not have much impact. Imagine living without the intensity of emotions – how lacking in passion and compassion life would be. It is the passion we each bring to life that ignites the holy fire within our hearts and the compassion for all creation that brings the highest human and spiritual qualities to the fore. A heart that aches also has the greatest capacity for joy.

> *"I can do all things through God who strengthens me."*
> *—The Holy Bible*

Every thought we think, every word we speak and every deed we perform has an effect on the whole. If we think negative thoughts, utter hurtful words or perform evil deeds, then by the law of cause and effect we will produce bad karma for ourselves.

We say, "What goes around comes around" and "We reap what we sow". This shows that the notion of karma (divine retribution in Hindu) is, at least subconsciously, firmly ensconced in the human psyche of the western world.

Every action provokes a reaction, and the polarities are constantly at work, producing a seemingly never-ending cycle of ups and downs, highs and lows.

This process is termed "bound to the wheel of karma" by the Buddhists, an apt description indeed.

> *"We are not punished for our sins,*
> *We are punished by our sins."*
> *—The Buddha*

How do we get off this merry-go-round? By realising that without knowing and experiencing the "bad", we cannot know the "good", that both are gifts from God and that both need to be transcended to achieve balance, or equilibrium.

"When we have learned to act from pure love and react to all people and situations equally with pure love, then we have released ourselves from the wheel of karma. We have reached self-liberation and the light finally has transcended the dark."

We achieve this balance by reminding ourselves of who we are, namely, sparks of the divine, perfect beings created in God's image. This is our real essence – to which nothing can be added or taken away. It is the false self, the conditioned, needy self, that still looks for approval from the outside world, that laps up praise and then is thrown into despair and inner darkness when approval is withdrawn.

Praise and criticism are to be taken equally lightly and need not influence us or upset our equilibrium.

Giving the approval and love you crave to yourself and accepting yourself as you are at this moment in time, totally and unconditionally, is the lever which will lift you from the darkness into the light.

Manifesting with light

Once we have fully entered into the divine I AM THE I AM reality, we will be freed from all restrictions and energy blocks and in perfect, divine health on all levels of our being. We will then experience ourselves as one with God, knowing at the same time we are self-realised individuals.

We will become part of the universal love and light of God.

When we are fully aligned with the divine will our inspiration will come directly from our divine God-self and thus our mind and emotions will be divinely guided also. The light of God will travel through the layers of our being from the spiritual layer, to the mental layer, the emotional and finally into the densest layer, the physical body, where it will manifest perfectly, just as God has intended.

We will then allow love=light to nourish us mentally, inducing a love for all sentient beings, and emotionally, resulting in feelings of peace, fulfilment and harmony. The light will flow through us uninterrupted by negative mental or emotional programming, free from any energy blocks.

We will attain balance on all levels and universal light will flow freely through us.

We will radiate love and light and by the law of attraction, we will now attract more love and light into our lives.

We will each be a perfect image of our Creator; the Creator and the created will have become ONE!

"Perfection is reached, not when there is no longer anything to add,
but when there is no longer anything to take away."
—Antoine de Saint-Exupery

This is the reality we are busy creating at present. It is a work in progress.

At the moment however, we maybe ill-at-ease or even experiencing "dis-ease".

From the level of light, all "dis-ease" arises from the notion that we are separate from God, the source of unconditional love. Lost, we have travelled through lifetimes looking for love in places where it can never be found, namely, outside ourselves, and on our journeys, we have picked up many different negative beliefs, most of which we are still holding on to. Negative beliefs produce negative emotions, and negative emotions if they persist over longer periods of time will eventually result in physical "dis-ease". The energy starts off as light and love from God but being hindered in its flow and not allowed to express itself freely, becomes distorted and more and more dense, producing energy blocks which eventually manifest into physical reality. It is these blocks in our energy field that we need to release so that we become joyful, happy and healthy and have the perfect body-shape.

> *"Turn your face to the sun*
> *and the shadows fall behind you."*
> —*Maori proverb*

Wheels of light: the chakras

As light=love is the universal energy, which has created and is at present sustaining us, it therefore is also the energy available to us for releasing the energy blocks, which are preventing us from being healed and achieving our highest potential.

In this section, we'll endeavour to dissolve these energy-blockages through connecting to God and channelling light into the chakras and the layers of the auric field. At the same time, we'll connect to mother earth, via our foot chakras in order to ground ourselves and then draw nourishing energy from her.

Please note that energy work should never be attempted under the influence of alcohol or other mind or mood altering substances.

The chakras – energy centres of the body

Most commonly it is taught that the human body contains seven major psychic centres, termed chakras, (derived from the Sanskrit, meaning "wheels of light").

In Fig. 1 (p.58) you will see the seven major chakras plus two minor ones the foot and palm chakras. The traditional location of each chakra correlates with a major gland, or glands, and a main autonomic nerve plexus within the body. Each chakra energetically feeds the physical body, connecting via the glandular system, and so affecting the workings and the health of the whole body. Healers and psychics with a background in psychotherapy or counselling have also observed that the point where each chakra is located corresponds with the points in the body where psychosomatic illness most commonly manifests.

The chakras are moving, whirling vortexes of energy, each rotating at a different speed and therefore creating a different vibratory rate, or frequency. This vibratory rate is psychically perceived as a colour. Colour, as energy, arises from the subtle interaction between darkness and light. Colour is light, broken down into wavelengths, into different vibratory rates. Violet, having the shortest wavelength has the fastest vibratory rate, or highest frequency. Red, having the longest wavelength, has the slowest vibratory rate. White light contains all the colours of the spectrum. The colours traditionally assigned to the chakras are the colours of the rainbow. In ascending order the chakras are:

NUMBER	COLOUR	NAME	LOCATION	PLEXUS & GLAND
1	Red	Base	Tailbone or coccyx	Pelvic plexus, Gonads
2	Orange	Sacral	Womb, lower abdomen	Hypogastric plexus, Adrenals
3	Yellow	Solar Plexus	Just above waist line	Solar plexus, Pancreas
4	Green	Heart	Mid-chest	Cardiac plexus, Thymus gland
5	Blue	Throat	Throat	Pharyngeal plexus, Thyroid gland
6	Indigo	Third eye	Centre of brow	Nasociliary plexus, Pituitary gland
7	Violet	Crown	Top of head	Cerebral, Pineal gland

Each of these perpetually rotating wheels of light creates an energy vortex that draws the light=love of God (the source, or universal energy field), together with very important sunlight, into the physical body via the subtle bodies (the mental, emotional and spiritual bodies) that make up the aura.

One of the cosmic laws states "As above, so below". In order to achieve a balanced energy field, the incoming energy from above – the heavenly energy – needs to be balanced with the incoming energy from mother earth. (A process where earth energy enters the auric field/chakra system via the foot chakra) This process is commonly known as grounding and many highly spiritually developed people are not grounded, as their being dwells too much in the lofty realms of heaven.

This is not a good state of affairs, and can actually affect our health, a fact into which we will go in more detail later on in the chapter.

The chakras are multi-functional, containing emotional, creative and celestial components and as we consciously allow more and more light=love to flow into the chakras, blockages of an emotional, mental or physical nature are cleared.

A healthy chakra in working order will be open and spinning clockwise, thus drawing energy from the universal energy field into itself.

If we are completely aligned with the divine will of God, energy will flow through us freely and the chakras will be in perfect working order. Sadly, for most of us this is, as yet, not the case. If we are presently not in the divine flow, which allows our lives to go smoothly and without interruption, we will be currently encountering negativity on our path. We may react to unpleasant experiences by blocking our feelings and stopping a great deal of the natural energy flow, at times even cutting ourselves off from the source, the light and love of God. (When this happens we may say "I feel so cut off" another example of spiritual truth reflected in day-to-day language). If for instance, we've been disappointed by a loved one, we may block the energy in our heart centre, so stopping ourselves from experiencing any more emotional pain, as we've not yet developed the art form of loving unconditionally,

This form of denial will slow the energy flow in our heart and finally create an energy block in the heart chakra. If we stay "heavy hearted", this may eventually result in a physical heart problem. If a friend deeply disappoints us and we feel we cannot possibly speak out, we may acquire a blockage in the throat chakra and this may result in a physical problem, such as a sore throat. The same process applies to all of the chakras.

If we block out negative experiences and do not find a successful way to deal with them, finally healing and releasing them, we will in turn create energy blocks in our chakras. Our chakras will become clogged up and blocked with the negative, stagnant energy. They may eventually start to spin irregularly or counter-clockwise, which will direct the energy flow out of the physical body, thus interfering with the metabolism. This is why, in cases of shock, the spin of the crown and/or third eye chakra becomes reversed and we very often feel dizzy. In the case of severe dis-ease the chakras might even become distorted and, at its worst, torn.

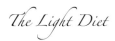

The aspects and functions of the chakras

1ST CHAKRA, THE BASE CHAKRA:

This chakra is the seat of desire and of the will to live and survive. It is the root of all growth and awareness of human divinity. The aspects of this chakra relate to physical survival: food and shelter, eating and sleeping and also the "fight or flight" reaction. The base chakra is the seat of the vital energy force, or creative energy (termed Kundalini in Sanskrit). When we are well grounded and the life-force is flowing fully through this centre, we will have a strong will and a zest for life.

If the incoming life-force is blocked, we will be ungrounded, "not present", and will spend a lot of the time asleep and be generally low in energy, often with an absence of physical strength and stamina and not much interest in the outside world. At its worst we can even lose our will to live.

2ND CHAKRA, THE SACRAL CHAKRA:

The aspects of this chakra relate to procreation and love for the family. It is also the centre where the first spark of inspiration to create is ignited. If this centre functions well, the giving and receiving of sexual and physical pleasures will be balanced, we will enjoy both. If the centre is blocked, we will be lacking in sex drive and general vitality. Also the impetus to create will be stifled or absent.

3RD CHAKRA, THE SOLAR PLEXUS CHAKRA:

The aspects of this chakra relate to the ego, the identity we seek to develop in this life, therefore it is sometimes called "the mind in the stomach". The questions of "Who am I? Why am I here? Where do I come from?" arise from this chakra. If we feel strong in our identity, we will feel connected with our soul brothers and soul sisters and the universe at large and furthermore will be emotionally peaceful and content, rising happily to life's challenges. One of the main functions of this chakra is the right use of personal power, its negative aspect being the abuse of power.

If the solar plexus chakra is not functioning properly, fear and anxiety can overcome us producing feelings of insecurity and isolation. If this chakra is closed, we will block our feelings, perhaps even deadening them. The solar plexus chakra is the highest of the three lower chakras (i.e., the base, the sacral and the solar plexus chakras) and serves as a connection to the central chakra, the heart, the seat of love. At present, society as a whole still operates from the point of the negative aspects of the solar plexus chakra, namely, fear, anxiety and power abuse. In order to compensate for those fearful emotions, willpower, and force are applied. However, many of us are now making the transition to acting in accordance with the divine higher will, from your heart-chakra, overcoming fears which are directly related to the "death of the lower ego self", which is frightened of losing its false identity.

4ᵀᴴ Chakra, the Heart Chakra:

The aspects of this chakra are love and the attainment of balance between the three higher and the three lower chakras.

It provides the link between our physical and spiritual aspects.

This centre is the seat of love and compassion for nature, all sentient beings and creation. If this centre is open, we will be able to perceive the good and bad in everything and everyone without attachment or criticism, and we will have the capacity to love ourselves unconditionally. Faith is one of the motivating forces, coupled with the striving for balance on all levels of existence.

As the heart centre connects to the throat centre, it is important for us to make an effort to communicate with love, to speak from the heart.

If this chakra is not functioning well, we will find it difficult to give unconditional love, always needing something in return. If the heart centre shuts down altogether, a heart attack or similar problem may result.

5ᵀᴴ Chakra, the Throat Chakra:

The aspects of this chakra are knowledge and expression of the self and the ability to communicate this to the world on all levels of being. If this chakra is working well, we are happy in our chosen profession or life's work and are able to express our creativity in a way that is naturally joyful to us.

This chakra is the link between the material (the body chakras) and cosmic consciousness (the head chakras), and once we are firmly established within ourselves – free of the attachments to the world and master of our total self – it will lead us towards the true birth of our divine self.

A blocked throat chakra, signifies a fear of failure, of not being able to realise our dreams. (that is, of being unable to bring the dreams of the head chakras through into the material realm of the body chakras). We can then become insecure, holding ourselves back in order to prevent disappointment to ourselves or others. Often this behaviour spirals into a victim-consciousness, closing the energy centre down even further.

6ᵀᴴ Chakra, the Third Eye Chakra:

The aspects of this energy centre are insight and intuition. Memories are also stored here along with the dreams and visions we have for our lives. This chakra is the seat of all psychic and clairvoyant abilities and is linked to the way we understand and process mental concepts. If this chakra is working well we will be able to create our own reality in harmony with universal laws and project outward into our lives what we desire.

This chakra is where negative and positive, the components of duality, become balanced, bringing with it a sense of oneness, so that we realise we're spiritual beings, having a human experience.

When this chakra is blocked, we can become mentally confused by negative belief systems or held back by binding agreements made in this or previous lives. A blockage in this centre often leads to "psychic headaches" because we do not allow our ideas to flow freely, often becoming highly self-critical.

7ᵀᴴ Chakra, the Crown Chakra:

This centre is the seat of higher consciousness and provides the link to the source, the light=love of God. If this centre is developed and open, we will be aware of our spirituality and will have integrated it into our mental, emotional and spiritual life.

This is the centre where finally the illusion of the individual self is dissolved and enlightenment, or self-illumination, is attained. When this happens, we are able to achieve liberation from the wheel of karma, finally realising our own divinity.

If this chakra is closed, we will have no concept of spirituality, nor will we be aware of our true nature.

The Two Palm and Foot Chakras:

The palm and foot chakras are of great importance, as they are small force-centres through which energy passes. The foot chakras provide a connection with the earth, so that positive energy, derived from mother earth, can be taken up into the body, while accumulated negative energy can be released.

The Human Energy Field or Aura:

The human energy field emanates from, and surrounds, the physical body. It is a living, pulsating energy and can be described as luminous, radiating a variety of colours. As it spins, each chakra produces its own electromagnetic field. This field then combines with fields generated by the other chakras to produce the auric field.

The aura provides "the space" which contains our emotional, thought, memory and behavioural patterns, all of which are living energies, vibrating at different rates. For instance, the lighter our thoughts are, the lighter the vibration and colour in our aura. If we think heavy thoughts, the vibration will effectively "sink" and slow down.

The aura is comprised of seven interpenetrating subtle bodies (Fig.2), each vibrating at a different rate, giving rise to a different colour. The rate of vibration is slowest at the densest level, the physical level, and becomes quicker and therefore lighter and brighter, as it rises up through the ever-more subtle levels. This vibrational matrix forms the human energy field, which may become stronger or weaker, brighter or duller, depending on the physical, emotional and spiritual health and awareness of the individual.

If we are very angry, the colour red, the lowest of the colour vibrations visible in the auric field, will show up. This can be perceived by a sensitive person and now also measured scientifically by analysing recorded wave patterns with the help of an oscilloscope. The phenomena of being able to perceive the colours of the auric field is known to mankind in general, albeit mostly on a subconscious level. Where else would the metaphor, "I'm seeing red" if we are very angry, come from?

The health and brightness of the aura is affected by weather patterns; for instance, a prolonged lack of sunshine will dull the colours of the auric field. Also if we suffer an accident or shock, it will show up as distorted patterns in our auric field. Drugs of any kind, which includes alcohol and cigarettes, leave the aura looking grey and, to a healer's hands, feeling sticky. I have surprised many a client during a spiritual healing session by telling them which drugs they had indulged in the previous night.

Beyond the aura are evermore-subtle collective bodies, which eventually merge into the universal energy field, into the light, God, the Source of all that is. It is this which connects and interpenetrates everything, on every level of existence.

The term "loving ourselves" considered from the highest vantage point, the point of light, really mean that we are inviting the light of God into our personal energy field; thus surrendering ourselves completely to God's love.

The amount of God's unconditional love we are able to take in equates to the amount of love we are able to feel for ourselves.

Most often, the problem doesn't lie with the giving of love, as we possess a good heart, but with the receiving of God's love, due to feelings of lack of self-worth and other related issues. These are the exact thought-forms and emotional patterns stored in the aura.

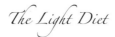

The light connection: a 5-step process

To be able to consciously connect with the divine, heavenly light of God and start the "light-work" of clearing our mental and emotional blockages, we will need to first go through a light-connection process, which consists of five steps.

1)   Aligning with God's divine will and purpose

2)   Aligning with the earth energies – grounding

3)   Aligning with the heavens – attunement

4)   Closing down the chakras and protecting the auric field

5)   Giving thanks

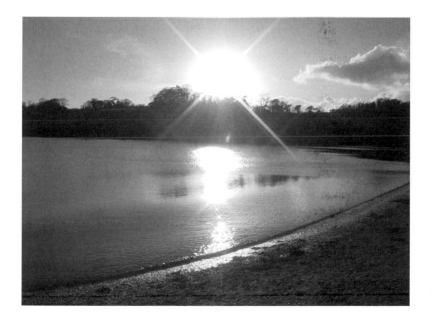

STEP 1: ALIGNING WITH GOD'S DIVINE WILL AND PURPOSE

If you are planning to take a shower, you step into the cubicle and make sure that you stand right underneath the showerhead, don't you? The same is also true if we would like to be aligned with the light of God; we step "out of the way of the ego and into the path of light".

We've already ascertained that God, being unconditional love in action, only has the highest purpose for us at heart. God's sole wish is that we become like Him, namely, pure love and light in action. This can only be achieved when we are happy and contented with our lot in life. The path to achieving just that is the one God presently is endeavouring to guide us on to.

However, our mental and emotional conditioning may tell us otherwise. Deep inside we cannot conceive an all-encompassing love, devoid of judgment and criticism, which has only our highest good for its aim. And rather than following God's guidance in accordance with His divine will, the little self, acting from the ego, kicks in, to make up for our lack of trust, faith and patience in God. As we can't wait for the manna from heaven we impatiently take matters into our own hands, forging ahead to pursue our fortune, forgetting that what seems like a good prospect might not be so in the long run. Remember, only God has the overview; He is the divine director of our lives and has the divine plan for our salvation in hand.

To be open to receiving all the riches God has to offer, we have to allow our ego to step out of the way first, by deciding firmly that we now will follow the motto – "Let go, let God!"

To manifest with the light of God, we have, first and foremost, to become aligned with God's divine will, which is identical to our own divine higher will. However, the lower ego is constantly trying to assert itself as an entity separate from God. It is literally fighting to the death, for it fears its annihilation, which it knows will come one day soon. What the frightened ego does not understand is that only its lower qualities, such as fear, greed and lust are to be transformed, but that it will still exist in its own right as part of the whole.

The ego's fear of losing control, by handing over power to a seemingly unknown outside force, can at times be totally overwhelming and, at its worst, downright crippling.

The ego will resort to any trick in the book, to all the negative programming, patterning and conditioning it has ever received, to ensure that we hang on to our own false identity, to that which keeps us separate from God and our true I AM THE I AM conscious state of being.

In order to align with God's divine will and purpose it is necessary to let go of all that is not love and any other unhealthy attachments and expectations.

Affirm the following; first out loud three times, followed by affirming six further times in your mind.

(Try to put as much passion as possible behind these affirmations, as this will speed up the energy process. Please ask God, your guardian angel and the healing angels to give you a hand.)

LETTING GO AFFIRMATIONS:

"I am consciously letting go of all that is not Love in my life.

I am consciously letting go of anything that is not in my highest purpose.

I am consciously letting go of anything which is not in my highest truth.

I am consciously letting go of anything which is not in my highest integrity.

I am consciously letting go of any expectations I have from people, situations or life as a whole.

I am now ready to allow God to give me the riches that are for my highest good and the highest good of all sentient beings on this planet.

And so be it!

And so be it!

And so be it!"

Now you are ready for the actual alignment with God's divine will and divine plan. It helps to also affirm an alignment with God's divine timing for you. This process is best done in the morning immediately upon awakening, before any negative thoughts are able to sneak in. If practised on a daily basis, these powerful affirmations will affect a real shift in your life, that is the shift from functioning from your lower ego, or little self, to operating from your higher divine self, which is identical with God. Over the years, many of my clients and workshop participants, having practised these affirmations, experienced major life-transformations as a direct outcome of this spiritual practice.

Again, please put your heart and soul into these affirmations, as this will show you wonderful results much faster.

Affirm the following out loud three times first, and then in your mind for another six times in the morning.

DIVINE ALIGNMENT AFFIRMATIONS:

"I am aligning my will with God's divine will.

I am aligning myself with God's divine purpose.

I am aligning myself with God's divine plan.

I am aligning myself with God's divine laws.

I am aligning myself with God's divine timing.

I AM THE I AM.
I AM THE I AM.
I AM THE I AM.
And so be it!
And so be it!
And so be it!"

Thank God and the angels for the help you have received.

By faithfully repeating these affirmations from your heart you will soon feel an increased energy flow and a greater sense of well-being and connectedness. This will have a beneficial effect on your mental, emotional and physical health, and change your life for the better in many unexpected, beautiful ways.

Step 2: Aligning with the earth energies – grounding

To balance the incoming heavenly light vibrations, we need to be firmly grounded in mother earth and strive to achieve what I term "integrated spirituality", where we, the beings of light dwelling in a physical body, partake consciously of life on earth in a balanced spiritual, mental, emotional and physical manner. Even some spiritually highly developed people can have an unbalanced approach to life: they can become disinterested in the physical aspects of their lives, deeming them to be of no importance; they may even find certain aspects of physical life simply "non-spiritual". This premise is a great misunderstanding, as to fully function on this earth plane, to be able to fulfil our divine mission here on earth, we have to be fully present in body, mind and spirit. This means we cannot escape living, and unfortunately suffering, by avoiding life and escaping into the higher realms of spirit.

Self-illumination means, just as the term suggests, that we have illuminated all the aspects of the self – the lower spiritual, the mental, the emotional and the physical aspects – and that the light has penetrated through all the layers of our being. If we don't participate in life fully, experiencing the shadow side of life and our very being, we cannot become enlightened, as there would be nothing to enlighten! Once we've become conscious of the dark and have allowed God, the light, to come into our lives, then the process of self-illumination can begin.

Everything is divine and the divine is in everything!

Now back to the subject of grounding. Before embarking on any energy work, such as bringing in the light through colour breathing or guided visualisations, we need to be properly grounded, rooted energetically into mother earth. This will give us a firm footing, so that we will be able to receive the incoming heavenly energies without becoming unbalanced and so that any excess energy has somewhere to discharge.

This concept is similar to the earth wire on all electrical appliances.

The most effective way to ground ourselves is by imagining that we are growing golden roots from the soles of our feet, allowing them to grow through some of the earth's layers until we feel firmly anchored. If we need extra strong grounding for high- level energy work, we can send the roots deeper into the earth until we arrive at the earth's core, where we will find a huge fossilised tree trunk. We can then wrap our roots firmly around this ancient, sturdy tree trunk for extra-strong grounding. Our roots, are, of course, hollow, as all roots are, so they can also serve as channels for energy running up into the foot chakras from mother earth and energy running down from the body, via the foot chakras, into mother earth.

Once the energy process is completed, we take our golden roots up through the layers of the earth or, if we have used the fossilised tree trunk method, unwrap our roots from the tree trunk first and then bring them up through the layers of the earth.

It is a good idea to be grounded at all times, so we can leave our golden roots just a few inches in mother earth permanently.

Mother earth, in unconditional service to humankind, will not only absorb our discharged negative energy but will also transmute it into positive "earth light".

This act of "grounding" is an energy process. The following exercise is an example of how to simply and successfully ground yourself (for instance after meditating, after experiencing a shock or after too many hours in front of the computer, which can also make you feel light-headed).

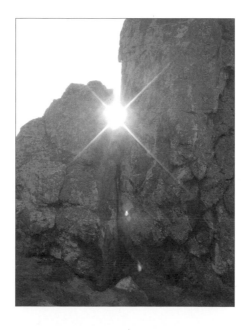

GROUNDING EXERCISE

Sit, with your back straight and your feet planted flat on the floor. (Remove your shoes if possible, though it's not absolutely necessary). Rest your outstretched arms, with your palms facing downward on your knees.

Now take a few deep breaths, breathing in light and love and releasing negativity on the out-breath.

After your breathing has slowed down, start to imagine golden roots sprouting from the soles of your feet – your foot-chakras. (See Fig. 1 the chakra drawing, p.XX) Visualise them, first growing through the floor of your room, then down through the foundations of your house and further down through the layers of the earth. Imagine each layer of earth becoming denser as your roots travel from the topsoil, down into the rocky layers of mother earth. Once your roots have arrived at the rocky layers, you can leave them there, firmly anchored in the ground.

Carry on breathing in love and light and releasing anything that is not love on the out-breath, until you feel more balanced and stable.

You may then draw your roots out of the deeper layers of the earth and just leave them in a few inches for the rest of your day.

Upon completions of this energy process, thank mother earth for allowing you to use her for your personal benefit and for all the love and nurturing she so freely bestows on you.

If you have the sensation of feeling light-headed after doing energy work, or indeed at any other time during the day, then further grounding may be necessary.

This can be achieved by a variety of means, a selection of which are outlined below:

1)   Taking food or water will often help you to be more grounded: drink mineral water and have a little chocolate or honey, a piece of bread or other carbohydrates which you are able to digest quickly to give your blood sugar level a quick boost. If you are doing a lot of energy work, I would advise you to eat pasta, potatoes or similar foods, which will have a grounding effect, during the day.

2)   Physical exercise will help you to ground yourself: running, walking, gardening and dancing are some activities that will help you to stay grounded.

3)   Gifts from mother earth will assist you: holding a piece of tree bark, especially from an oak tree, holding a large pebble or placing a haematite crystal in your pocket or, if you are able to do so, hugging a tree will greatly assist you in grounding yourself.

4)   Taking a nap and sleeping for about one hour will ground and refresh you.

5)   A long shower also has a good grounding effect.

STEP 3: ALIGNING WITH THE HEAVENS – ATTUNEMENT

During most of the energy work in this book we will be taking in light from above (the source, God, the universal energy field,) on the in-breath and releasing the negative energies which need clearing, on the out-breath, through our golden roots into mother earth.

As we breathe, prana, divine life-force, flows into the body. It's very important to learn to breathe properly, as breathing has a direct effect on life span; the slower and deeper we breathe, the longer we live!

As our physical, mental or emotional conditions change, so does our rate of breathing. If we are angry or frightened, breathing becomes fast and shallow; while during deep sleep, it becomes slow and regular. An average human breathes (one inhalation, one exhalation) thirteen to fifteen times a minute, which means that the body breathes 21,000 to 21,600 times in a twenty-four hour cycle.

The faster we breathe the more energy the body uses, taking away valuable life force in the process. If we are able to maintain a normal breathing rate of not more than fifteen breaths per minute, or if we can slow down our breathing rate even more, we can conserve energy, increase our level of vitality and also, very importantly, live longer.

FULL BREATH EXERCISE

The completed breath consists of three parts, which will flow together as one movement on the in-breath. On the out-breath lower the shoulders, contract the ribs and push in the abdomen.

a) *Abdominal*

Place your hands lightly on your abdomen. Now think of a balloon to be filled and totally emptied and exhale. Breathe in slowly through your nose and now feel your hands spreading apart and separating. Exhale slowly through your mouth, feel yourself emptying completely.

b) *Intercostal*

Place your hands lightly on your ribcage, imagining your ribs as an accordion.
Exhale through your mouth. Now inhale slowly through your nose and feel your ribs expanding; then exhale through your mouth again and let go.

c) *Clavicular*

Take short puffs to operate the upper section of the lungs.

CLEANSING BREATH EXERCISE

This breath might be simple, but it is very effective:

a)   *Inhale a complete, full breath.*

b)   *Retain the air for a few seconds.*

c)   *Now pucker your lips, as if you want to whistle, and exhale some of the air with vigour.*

d)   *Then pause for a moment, holding the (remaining) breath.*

e)   *Now exhale a little more air and repeat until the air is completely exhaled.*

Relaxation, meditations and other forms of energy work will further enhance the process of slowing down and deepening your breathing.

The all important requirement, for every breathing exercise is, that you firmly state the following intent:

> **"I am breathing in love and light and when I breath out
> I release and let go of all that is not love."**

You might want to repeat this phrase in your mind as you are practising this exercise.

With your breath flowing gently and rhythmically, you can now use it to bring in the light of God.

As you ask from your heart for God's light to enter you, the divine universal energy will flow into your personal energy field by entering the top of your head, through the crown chakra. It will flow through your chakras and auric field all the way down to your feet and finally through your foot chakras into mother earth, taking with it any stagnant negative energies which had previously created energy blocks in your aura and chakras.

In effect, attunement is the first step on the ladder of your healing process of cleansing, clearing and releasing the negativity that has held unwanted mental, emotional and physical patterns – including the body-shape you are unhappy with – in place in your energy field up until now.

The following is a lovely, highly effective attuning exercise:

DIVINE LIGHT ATTUNEMENT

Begin by grounding yourself by growing golden roots. (As explained earlier.)

Breathe in love and light and feel those energies surrounding you.

Relax and let go on the out-breath.

Now breathe in peace, and sense the energy of peace within your heart.

Release and let go of any worries you may have on the out-breath.

With every breath you take, the energy of love and light surrounding you becomes stronger and stronger.

Imagine that the energy of God surrounds and protects you.

Now visualise the top of your head, your crown chakra, like a beautiful rosebud, which is slowly opening its petals with every breath of love and light you take.

Soon you are able to feel the light of God, which is all around you, flowing into your crown chakra and from there the divine energy gently flows all the way through your energy centres, sweeping away any psychic debris on its path. The murky energy flows out through your foot chakras and is absorbed by mother earth.

Then gently imagine the petals of the rose closing again into a bud.

Keep your roots a few inches in the earth and give thanks to God and mother earth for their abundant love for you.

As with everything, it is practice that makes you perfect. Think of spiritual exercise as flexing a set of new muscles, muscles you have not used very much previously.

Walking to the shops on a daily basis does not make a marathon-runner, as you know. With regular practice you will be able to move from sensing the energies around you to actually physically feeling them, and in time, an exercise that previously would have taken you ten minutes to do will happen in an instant.

Also you will find that after some time of regular practice your whole being will start to crave these spiritual exercises, they will become effortless and a true joy to indulge in. A little bit like spiritual toffees, yum!

THE POWER OF VISUALISATION, OR GUIDED IMAGERY:

In conjunction with the sacred breath we will now use the power of visualisation, or guided imagery, in order to make the energy process even more potent. These energy processes are based on an important universal law:

"Energy follows thought".

We are all co-creators with God, who has given us the gift of a limitless mind, which we are free to utilise in creating and manifesting a positive reality through the use of guided imagery.

Visualisation is a creative process and takes place in the third eye chakra.

It may take a little time before you are able to see a colour, an image or a scene on your "inner screen", however that's quite normal and no cause for concern.

In fact some people who are not visually gifted, so to speak, will sense and sometimes even smell the energies instead.

The most important factor in this process is, that your "heart is in it" and that you put much positive intent behind what you would like to imagine. This passionate intent is the real spiritual rocket-fuel you need in order to manifest your desires.

In any manifestation process make sure that you "think with your heart" and the outcome will always be a good and a light one.

HOW TO IMPROVE YOUR VISUALISATION SKILLS

It's a very good idea to practise your visualisation skills with something easy. You might start by studying everyday objects around you in close detail. Take, for example, a vase; observe its shape, texture and colour. Then close your eyes and picture it as vividly as possible. Once you feel you are able to visualise it confidently, fill the vase with fragrant flowers, perhaps from your garden. Observe the flower filled vase; then close your eyes and picture the colour, texture and shape of the vase and flowers; you may even imagine their perfume.

With some practice, when you close your eyes you will find it much easier to get a sense of an object or colour on your inner screen.

As colours seem to be difficult for many people to visualise, you might like to collect some colourful objects with which to practise your visualisation skills.

You might want to purchase a set of ribbons in the colours of the rainbow and practise with them. To visualise the colour gold, which is used a lot in guided imagery, as it is the universal healing colour, take a good look at a piece of golden jewellery and then close your eyes and "think gold".

It is important to not to try too hard; do not force anything. Simply allow these "spiritual muscles" to grow naturally in time with your practice.

Just as you are able to dream in colour, so you will soon be able to visualise in colour.

Even if you still find visualisation difficult, here is a simple, but beautiful meditation guaranteed to enhance your visual abilities.

CANDLE VISUALISATION

Make sure that you have ten minutes to yourself.

Place a simple white candle on a saucer in front of you, so that you can see it comfortably from where you will be sitting, then light it.

Sit down in a chair, with your back straight, your feet flat on the floor and your arms outstretched, with your palms facing upward in a receiving gesture, resting on your knees.

Now gaze in a gentle, relaxed way at the candle flame.

Notice what size and shape it is; also notice any colours within or surrounding the flame.

Allow about three minutes to do this and then close your eyes gently and allow the image of the candle to emerge on your inner screen.

How large is it? Does it flicker? What is the quality of its light?

You will probably notice that the image floats around. Just keep following it until it fades from view. When it does, simply open your eyes and gaze at the actual candle.

Again, allow three minutes of observation time.

Gaze gently at the flame; then close your eyes when you are ready.

Notice what you can see on your inner screen.

As before, keep following the 'inner flame' until it fades away.

Open your eyes and blow out the candle flame, sending the light out into the world as you do so.

This exercise is far more then "meets the eye". It will also have a deeply relaxing, calming effect on you and is a wonderful meditation in itself, if you take the subject of "light" further into contemplation while you gaze at the candle.

Enjoy your visualisations and they soon will flow beautifully!

STEP 4: CLOSING DOWN THE CHAKRAS AND PROTECTING THE AURIC FIELD

THE PRACTICE OF "CLOSING DOWN":

During spiritual practice your energy centres, your chakras, will open naturally in order to allow maximum light to enter your auric field, and at times special imagery can be added to aid this process. While your chakras are open, you will be extra sensitive to all incoming energies. This is fine for the duration of your energy work; however after completion of your spiritual practice, if the chakras were to be left open, you could be subject to a variety of negative influences, which could make you feel ungrounded or even nauseated. Strong environmental influences, like radiation or severe, negative thought forms from other people could find their way easily into your energy field and leave you mentally disturbed and confused.

Please approach all energy work with an open heart and an open mind, but also with your intellect, your power of reasoning, intact. As a rule, if an exercise does not feel right to do or if, after practising it repeatedly, it still does not "go in", then let it go for the moment. It may be that this is the wrong kind of exercise for you or the timing might just not be right.

The term "closing down" seems to infer a complete closing down of operations of your chakras, but this is not the case. The chakras are, by the process of closing down, returned to everyday operating levels. Through the power of visualisation, you will create a protective energy filter around the chakras that will filter any negative energy out and allow only high vibrational love energy in.

There are a variety of closing down visualisations. Here is one that is very effective and easy to follow. Remember, as with all energy work, to ground yourself via your golden roots at the beginning of your spiritual exercise. Note also that the closing down always commences from the crown-chakra downwards through the rest of your chakras. The sequence is therefore as follows:

- Crown chakra
- Third eye chakra
- Throat chakra
- Heart chakra
- Solar plexus chakra
- Sacral chakra
- Base chakra

CLOSING DOWN PROCESS – THE ROSE

Imagine that your chakras are like deep-pink roses, whose petals are open.

Try to get a sense of this magnificent flower and visualise its beautiful, velvety, petals.

When you are ready, see the petals slowly closing until the rose resembles a tight rosebud.

Start this process with your crown-chakra, ending at the base-chakra.

To give extra protection, visualise a golden cross, surrounded by a golden circle, placed on top of each of the rosebuds.

Once your chakras are closed, draw up the golden roots, bringing them back through the layers of the earth and leave them just a few inches deep in the ground.

Always give thanks for the help you have received.

THE PRACTICE OF PROTECTING YOURSELF

As you are well aware, you are surrounded by a variety of negative influences at all times. These influences might be of an environmental nature, such as radiation from your mobile phone, computer or television. Furthermore you might live and work in an area of geopathic stress, which will also have a negative effect on your energy field. Also the negative influences might be of a psychic nature, such as people thinking of you in a harmful manner, and as a thought is an energy-packet, this will have a negative effect on your chakras and your auric field and might potentially drain your life-force, robbing you of your vitality.

Protection is only needed until you are fully present in the here and now of your divinity and you have become love, as divine love is the best possible protection available. However, this is not yet the case with most of humanity and therefore I would strongly recommend you to complete any spiritual exercises with some form of protection.

The following process is the one that I use most and has the extra benefit of leaving you, not only safely protected, but with a lovely, cosy feeling inside.

PROTECTION PROCESS – THE AURIC EGG

Imagine yourself to be like the egg-yolk inside an egg.

Now see beautiful, radiant golden energy filling the space where the egg white would be.

Imagine as much golden healing vibration around you as you like. (It does not matter if your egg becomes as large as an emu's egg!)

Then, in the place where you would normally find the eggshell, imagine a layer of strong electric blue, neon-bright energy.

Create this protective shell as thin or as thick as you like; it could go from several inches to several feet, both are absolutely fine.

Give thanks for the energies you have received.

I would strongly suggest that you not only protect your aura in this manner following spiritual exercises, but also every morning after your contemplations or meditations and every evening before going to sleep.

The routine of grounding, closing down and protecting yourself will be beneficial to you in situations where you find yourself emotionally, mentally or physically stressed and your energies are being eroded.

With practice, the whole process will only take minutes to implement, but will bring you a whole day of beneficial effects.

STEP 5: GIVING THANKS

A lways thank "the powers that be" for their cooperation after your spiritual practice, especially if you have asked angels, masters or guides for help.

Be mindful of the contribution mother earth makes to your life and well-being, and try to remember to show your gratitude to her for the services rendered to you, on a daily basis. The earth is not just a lump of soil; she is a living, breathing being, and an entity in her own right, with the name of Gaia, evolving just like you. As you are filling yourself with light, so mother earth is on her way to becoming a star.

Find below some "thank you" affirmations, which you might like to repeat:

GIVING THANKS AFFIRMATIONS

I give thanks to God for holding me in the palm of His hands.

I give thanks to the angels for being always by my side.

I give thanks to my guides and the masters of light for their support.

I give thanks to mother earth for giving herself to me unconditionally.

It would be beneficial to include these or other affirmations like them, in your morning contemplations or meditation routine.

In the chapters ahead we will be using colour-breathing, guided visualisations, inner journeywork and other energy processes to clear your chakras of any negativity, so that you may achieve, not only the perfect body-shape, but also the perfect life for you.

Please memorise the 5 step routine and apply it faithfully in your spiritual practice.

Step 1: Aligning with God's divine will and purpose:
You become ONE with God's will.
Step 2: Aligning with the earth energies – grounding:
You are safely anchored.
Step 3: Aligning with the heavens – attunement:
You are connected with the light.
Step 4: Closing down the chakras and protecting your auric field:
You are safe and protected.
Step 5: Giving Thanks
You are grateful for what you have received.

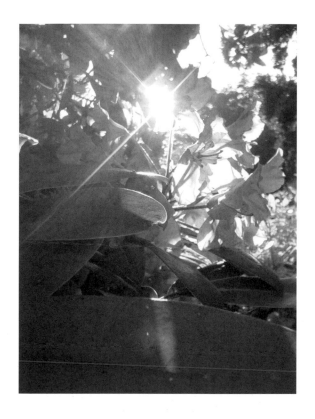

*"By meditation upon light and upon radiance,
knowledge of the spirit can be reached
and thus peace can be achieved."*
— Patanjali

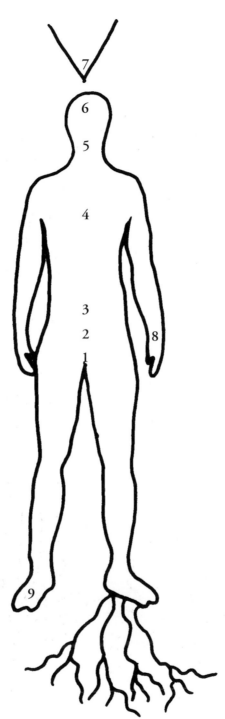

CHAKRA CHART (FIG. 1)

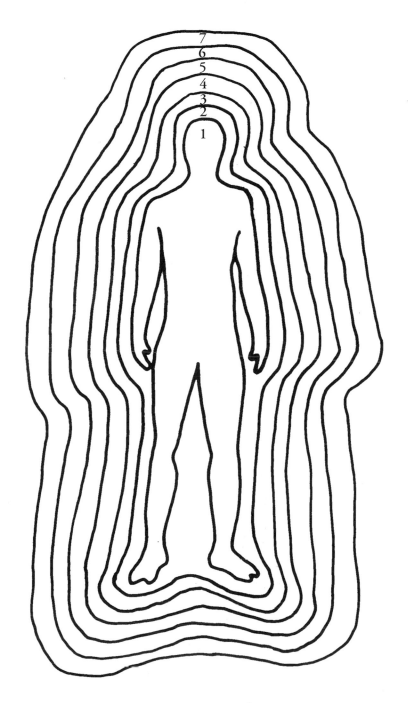

THE SEVEN LAYERS OF THE AURIC FIELD (FIG.2)

Part 4:
Mind matters

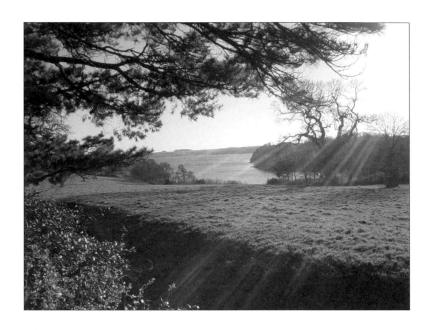

*"What we are today comes from thoughts of yesterday,
and our present thoughts build our life tomorrow.
Our life is the creation of our mind."*
—*The Buddha*

How what we think creates our reality

Our thoughts create our reality; this is the cosmic law that states "Energy follows thought" in action. The shape of our bodies and the state of the world around us exists as a reflection of our belief systems, which were put in place by the social, cultural and religious conditioning we received in this and any previous life times.

God has given us the power to create exactly what we need to experience, in order to find out who and what we truly are. We are each a divine spark clothed at present in a sheath of human thoughts and emotions, and a physical body. This divine spark, the soul is utilising the mind, the emotions and the body to learn to express its divinity.

To find out who we are, we have to experience, first hand, who we are not. We must realise, that we have created the darkness currently present in our lives, be it dark thoughts, dark emotions or dark situations, and that we have done this so that there is something for God's light to shine onto.

We have created negative thoughts, emotions and situations in order to be able to observe them and to learn from them. If we were to dwell in divine bliss from the day we were born, would we be able to appreciate this bliss, to know what it is, to know what it means and where it originated from? No, we would not and, most importantly, we would not be inclined to even ask the question. Why should we. We would be divine little bliss-bubbles, happily bobbing around in the world with no care or thought of anything else but ourselves. In short we would have no "self-awareness". Neither would we want any, as there would be no impetus, nothing outside of ourselves driving us to become aware. Self-awareness, of course, is the major ingredient in knowing who we truly are.

Only through suffering, through wanting to improve our lot, does humankind learn at this present time. (I do sincerely hope that we will soon be advanced enough to move from learning through suffering to learning through joy!)

When we suffer we start to ask ourselves questions, like "Why do I suffer? "What causes my suffering?" or "How can I stop suffering?" The pressure we receive from the outside world facilitates the process of our "looking within". Without these outside forces acting as a stimulus, our lives would be stagnant and stale. These truly are the forces of duality at play, and without this interplay, life on earth would cease to exist. Another extremely important aspect of our own suffering, as well as observing suffering in others, is that the emotional impact it has on us greatly facilitates the opening of our hearts to others and the world at large. How else would we be able to feel empathy, compassion and love for other people? A simple human caring about what is happening to our fellow soul-brothers and sisters has to be experienced before we are able to move to the notion of a higher, unconditional love for ourselves and others.

The world we see is the "out-pictured version" of our inner world. If our inner world is in turmoil, our outer world will be in turmoil too and we will perceive negativity everywhere. If our inner world is at peace, peace will be all around us and we will be able to perceive the good even in the worst situation.

And so our spiritual evolution moves forward; we will continue to experience duality, until there is no more need to do so and humankind has learned that love and kindness is all that's needed to live together in harmony on this lovely planet earth. The day will surely come where we will realise that wars are just an out-picturing of the lack of love, the fears, the internal wars, raging inside our own beings. When love and peace reign in every human heart, there will be peace and love on earth.

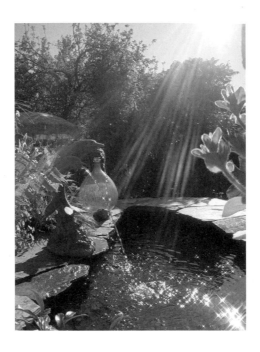

"Just as a picture is drawn by an artist,
surroundings are created by the activities of the mind."
—*The Buddha*

Owning the reality we have created

Just as we are each an aspect of the ONE, so is everything and everybody around us. All the things we like about our friends, relationships and the world at large and everything we dislike about the same are a direct reflection of what we like and dislike about ourselves.

"If you hate a person, you hate something
in him that is part of yourself.
What isn't part of ourselves doesn't disturb us."
—*Hermann Hesse*

We can be sure that, by courtesy of the universe, all that needs to be healed within us will be shown to us outside of ourselves through people, situations or circumstances which need the exact healing we require. This can, and mostly is, an unpleasant experience, as we do not enjoy being confronted with these aspects of ourselves. What we cannot stand about our neighbour down the road is something we deeply dislike within ourselves, something which needs to be healed.

Family and close friends often provide the greatest scope for healing and are therefore the ones we battle with frequently, as we are rarely prepared to see that the negative character traits our nearest and dearest display might in any way have anything to do with us or even, God forbid, be a reflection of what goes on inside us!

For most of us this is a truly frightening prospect to contemplate and takes some bravery to take on board. However, we will not be able to move forward with our lives until we begin to "own our stuff", i.e. the reality we are experiencing right now, and to see that every situation is of our own making (even though it may have taken several lifetimes to create).

Remember, that the present is just that, a present, a gift from God to you, for you to apply your power to choose right here, right now and make the changes you long for!

It is difficult and at times painful to accept that we have created the situations we find ourselves in and the negative states of body, mind or emotions or situations that accompany them. To be able to understand why we are in this predicament, we have to shift our viewpoint from ground zero to a higher level. We must start by endeavouring to see the bigger picture, by trying to see how life events have stacked up from past into present time. The bigger picture will, on reflection, show us that many unhappy situations have actually led to positive outcomes in the long run and have been of some benefit to ourselves or others. Of course, there is much suffering which from the human viewpoint does not make any sense at all, the reason being that we do not have the full overview. Can we trust that God's divine plan for us is in perfect order and that He has the divine, all-knowing overview for our highest purpose at heart? Can we trust that every tear we shed is for a very good reason and brings us closer to the truth of our divine self?

When we have truly taken responsibility for our lives, for the things we have thought, said or done in the past, and when we arc also honest with ourselves about what we feel right now in the present moment, we will really "own our stuff".

We will have moved on from the common practice of denial, a very widespread human disease, into acceptance of who we truly are in this moment. Then congratulations will indeed be due!

> *"Life is a sum of all your choices."*
> *— Albert Camus*

Once we take a good, honest look at ourselves, "warts and all", then a huge shift in awareness will begin to happen. We will become aware that the feelings we feel and the thoughts we think, and the emotions they make us feel belong to us and have nothing do to with anyone else, although they might of course, have been triggered off by an outside agency. Remember, no matter how other people might act towards us, it is our re-action to their behaviour that counts. We have the choice: will we respond with the "an eye for an eye, a tooth for a tooth" philosophy or are we going to ask ourselves the question "What would love do now?" and react accordingly?

The choice is ours and ours alone!

> *"If a man's mind becomes pure, his surroundings also become pure."*
> *— The Buddha*

Divine truth versus conditioned reality

When we are true to ourselves we are much more able to connect to the divine truth, which is the reality of all that IS.

All the wisdom we need is contained within the divine truth and once we are linked with our higher God-self, our mind will be anchored firmly in it.

> *"Truth is what the voice within tells you."*
> *— Mahatma Gandhi*

How do we find out what is the divine truth and what is not?

We do this by listening:

a) to our intuition, which is the voice of our soul (and the soul gets its information straight from the source, our higher God self) and

b) to what our body has to tell us. (When something "does not feel right", we can actually feel it in our solar plexus, the area around your navel.)

We need to be aware that the conditioned mind will try to throw a spanner into the works, as it will fervently resist change, not wanting to take any new concepts on board.

However, the more we as spiritual seekers are prepared to search for the truth, the more divine truth will be revealed to us.

> *"Truth is like a vast tree which yields more*
> *and more fruit the more you nurture it."*
> *— Mahatma Gandhi*

If we are not "in our truth" then we are "out of integrity". Integrity is the state of being whole, of being unified, integrated and in alignment with our highest good and our principles. Our body, mind, emotions and spirit then work in unison with the divine will. If we are in "full divine integrity", we will be incorruptible; we will no longer be swayed by any negative influences.

We will walk firm and steadfast on our chosen path.

Being in our truth means that we allow ourselves to communicate how we truly feel and what we really think about ourselves and the world at large. Of course our mind warns us not to do this, as previously the consequences of such actions have been far from positive. However, if we continue not being fully ourselves, we will attract more of the same negative situations towards us and go even deeper into denial of our divine nature.

Once we have learned to "speak our minds", we need to be mindful of how we communicate our truth. Although occasionally tough love has to be applied and the truth has to be used like a sword, most of the time the truth can be communicated in a gentle manner, without inflicting unnecessary hurt upon our soul brothers and sisters.

We would do well to develop what the Buddhists term the "art of harmlessness" towards all sentient beings and adopt a kind, considerate attitude towards the whole of creation, as "what goes round, comes round"!

To cement your alignment with the divine truth, use the following affirmations.

DIVINE TRUTH AFFIRMATION:

> **I am aligning my thoughts with the divine truth.**
> **I am aligning my words with the divine truth.**
> **I am aligning my actions with the divine truth.**
> **I am now in full alignment with the divine truth.**
> **I AM THE I AM.**
> **I AM THE I AM.**
> **I AM THE I AM.**
> **And so be it.**
> **And so be it.**
> **And so be it.**

Read these affirmations out loud three times and then repeat them in your mind a further six times, putting your heart and soul into it.

You might want to repeat these affirmations on a daily basis until you feel you have made the progress and shift you require.

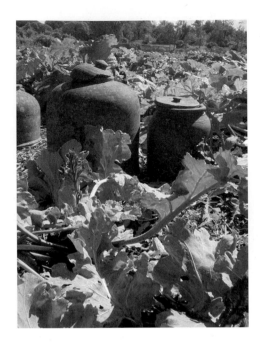

*"In the search for ultimate truth, if it fails to dawn on us,
it is we who have not found it.
Ultimate truth exists.
If we think deeply and reflect carefully,
we shall realise that we ourselves have our existence in ultimate truth."*
—His Holiness the Dalai Lama

How we have manifested our present reality

The reason why we do not perceive ourselves as "perfect" at present is because our minds have mis-created, they have created a "false reality" for us, which we have believed to be solid and real.

If our minds had been ONE with God at all times, we would now be perfect in His image, in body, mind and spirit.

Of course a long, long time ago, our mind was ONE with the divine mind. However, God realised that we had no awareness of our state as part of God and He therefore allowed us to descend into matter to give us the gift of finding out the true reality of our divine nature.

In order to do this successfully we were born with "spiritual amnesia" which made us forget our divine origin, a step necessary to spur our learning and search for truth. (This is the divine plan, lovingly designed by our creator God.) We also forgot that we are already perfect at the core of our being, that the body, mind and emotions had been given to us by God as learning devices, and that they are "illusions" in the sense of being subject to change and therefore not eternal, whereas the soul has eternal life and is indestructible.

So the soul journeys from lifetime to lifetime, bringing with it the sum-total of all its experiences into each new life, having acquired a host of false beliefs about itself, the nature of God and the world. Not having been in alignment with the divine truth for many lifetimes, the mind has created our present reality from the basis of its conditioned, human perception; a basis that is rooted in fear and lack of love. However this needed to be, given that we are learning who we truly are by experiencing who we are not.

Any creation of any sort that lacks love will be imperfect; therefore loving ourselves unconditionally is the most important ingredient in manifesting our desires (including our perfect body-shape).

So, the body, mind and emotions are just learning devices that enable us to become co-creators with God, thus facilitating our self-illumination. In essence there is only the self; we are each an identical part of the whole. What logically follows from this truth is that if we heal the mind, emotions and body completely, by releasing and healing all that is not love, we will not only return to our original divine state, but will greatly facilitate this process for the rest of the planet.

By the act of healing ourselves, we are healing those around us.

The medicine we need to take in ample measure is love, love, love – tons of unconditional love for ourselves – and the power of forgiveness that cures all ills. The spiritual, mental and emotional processes contained in this book are in fact "energy medicine". Energy medicine may taste bitter at times, but it is healing in the long run. Its application enable us to be in control of our destiny, allowing us to reclaim our power from outside sources and to instead rely on the power of light and wisdom that resides within our own being.

"We are what we think. All that we are arises with our thoughts.
With our thoughts we make the world."
—The Buddha

The process of creation

The act of creation first begins with a spark of inspiration. Once inspired, the mind forms a thought: an idea is born. If this idea is of interest, we may talk about it to someone, and if they think it's great too, we might put this idea, this thought, into practice. What has started off as a tiny spark of inspiration has now taken tangible form.

This is the act of creation and we all do this every day. (When you got up this morning didn't the "must have tea or coffee sign" flash up in your mind? You didn't need any advice on the matter; you just went to the kitchen and made the cup of tea or coffee and drank it.)

As a spark of inspiration descends into matter, it goes through various states of density. Such a spark of inspiration is very light in energy, especially if it is a lovely one. A thought is a lot denser than a spark; it vibrates at a lower frequency. (You will have walked into dense thought-forms before, as into a situation where people have been fighting or arguing.) Spoken words are denser still. (You are well aware of the devastating or immensely uplifting powers of the spoken word.) When we act on our inspiration we complete the act of creation.

In short the process of creation is: inspiration–thought–word–deed.

The quality of the inspiration and where it originates, determines the outcome of the creation. If the mind, the instrument by which we create, is inspired by thoughts of peace, love and light, we will create happy thoughts, speak loving words and perform, hopefully, many acts of random kindness. If we create something physical, whether it is a lovely supper or a new garment, it will sparkle with love and light. Anyone on the receiving end will be uplifted by eating the food we have cooked so lovingly or by looking at the lovely garment we've made.

Focusing and aligning the mind with our higher divine mind will ensure that we are divinely inspired and in perfect alignment with divine will, which equals our highest good.

Once firmly focused and aligned, the spark of light = love will lead to a loving thought and thus we are able to create the wonderful reality we so much desire.

At present however, our inspirations originate mainly from the denser regions of our being, namely from the conditioned mind. Our mind, clogged up and bogged down with false beliefs about ourselves, is not able to come up with truly uplifting stuff.

Quite the opposite, we tend to believe a number of negative things about ourselves.

We may even be convinced that we are failures, losers, inadequate, lazy, incompetent and downright selfish.

This has dire emotional consequences, the source and release of which we will deal with in the next chapter.

If we try to create from this distorted mind-set, which most of us are still trying to do, we will, quite logically, create a distorted reality.

Subject to the universal law of "like attracts like", we then will only attract more of the same experiences.

"He who sees all beings in his own self,
and his own self in all beings, loses all fear."
— The Upanishads

The effect of negative beliefs on body, mind and emotions

Deeply rooted negative beliefs tell us that there is not enough love, money, food, shelter and opportunity in this world, and that we cannot have what we want, as there just is not enough to go around.

Our minds dictate what we want from a position of lack within ourselves.

This feeling of lack within is the true state of the self and attracts more lack to itself,

The outcome is that we attract more lack, more want and more need, as negative states attract more negativity to themselves.

So, the thought "I want a perfect body" will just increase our feelings of not being perfect with the result that we will get more and more angry and frustrated at ourselves, hating our physique even more. Needless to say, the same goes for all our other wants and needs.

Our beliefs around food are particularly distorted. Conditioned by (nine times out of ten) the media, or possibly by dieting relatives, we may believe that certain foods have specific effects on us, most of them fattening.

It is the belief we have in these false "truths" which makes us either pile on the weight, or lose weight, not the actual food we eat. The body has no choice but to follow the commands of the mind, which is instructing it with negative thoughts about food.

What we think about the food we eat is the important thing.

It is not the food that is either fattening or slimming, as the case may be, but the beliefs you attach to the food!

Most of us, know at least one person who says that they can eat what they want and never either lose or put on any weight, which is perfectly true they simply don't.

Why? Because they firmly believe they won't!

Their belief that "I can eat what I want, when I want and stay the same weight" is enough to make their truth a reality.

The reason why a diet works for us is because we believe in it. We tell ourselves that this will work and for a short while it does… so why do we always seem to slip up?

It is, because we have not discovered the cause of our weight problem.

Once we have unearthed the negative belief that is the underlying cause of any problem, may it be mental, emotional or physical, it can be healed.

One of the most potent healing aids to rid ourselves of negative beliefs and replace them with positive ones, is the positive affirmation. Through the power of positive affirmations we can literally re-programme the mind and body, replacing negative thought forms or negative belief patterns, with positive ones, thus creating **lasting** results.

I would urge you to actually write out the positive affirmations from this point on. Writing things down means that you really mean business; you truly want to manifest your new, glorious reality. Write each affirmation down nine times at any session, nine being the number of completion. Of course, each time you write a positive affirmation your mind will immediately bring up a negative thought – a blocking-device. Compile a list of these. (Ruled notepaper works best and I suggest that you use different coloured pens, which will help to highlight the results visually) Begin by writing the positive affirmation on the left-side of the page, then, on the right-side, jot down the response that comes to your mind (most likely some form of denial). Write out your responses quickly, as this helps to unlock your subconscious mind, which is trying to hold on to its negative conditioning.

Keep on writing the same affirmations over and over again, until your negative responses turn into positive ones. When that has been achieved, you can continue with just the positive affirmations until you feel that the desired effect has been achieved. You will then have successfully re-programmed your conscious and subconscious mind in a positive manner and have achieved your goal.

Here are some key self-acceptance affirmations, you need to work with as often as possible, and please try to remember, "What you resist, persists".

Self- acceptance affirmations:

I, ___(your name) _____ , *accept my body.*

I, _____ , *accept my thoughts.*

I, _____ , *accept my feelings.*

I, _____ , *accept myself completely and unconditionally.*

JUST TO REMIND YOU AT THIS POINT:

The diet you need to follow is one that is **full of light and free of negativity!**

• **Your thoughts + beliefs create your reality.**

• **Positive thoughts + beliefs will create a positive reality.**

• **Negative thoughts + beliefs will create a negative reality.**

The more positive your thoughts and beliefs are, the lighter you will become in body, emotions, mind and spirit!

We may think that we have power over the mind, but we soon discover that the mind rules us; the mind is like a wild horse running away with us (a very apt Buddhist description).

In order to be able to create the reality we would like to create,
we need to tame the mind first.

To tame the mind, we need to examine its unruly contents. By close observation the negative beliefs, which are stopping us from achieving what we want and from being who we want to be in this precious lifetime, will come to light and can then be released and healing take place.

However, if we do not observe the mind in the spirit of unconditional self-acceptance and love, the negative thoughts will simply hide away, just as a child will hide if it has been caught doing something naughty. The mind will cooperate with us, only if the unwilling thoughts are coaxed out, like little foxes hiding in their underground burrow. These thoughts may have been suppressed for a long time, some of them most likely since early childhood. They have slipped into the subconscious mind and the subconscious will not give up and spew out its content easily for fear of retribution. This fear can stop any progress we could make. There is only one cure for this fear. It is to apply the energy medicine: unconditional love and complete positive self acceptance.

The only way to find out what is happening in the conscious mind and what is lurking in the subconscious is by spending time observing our thought-patterns, which we are normally not consciously aware of. This is a very important mental and spiritual practice and will bring great rewards.

"The most terrifying thing is to accept oneself completely."
—C. G. Jung

Set aside about ten minutes for this exercise at first and then increase the time-span to up to one hour, if you can.

Have pen and paper ready, to note down repetitive, persistent thought-forms, as they are the ones you will need to release first and foremost.

The best way to become the observer (which is a little tricky, as your mind is trying to control you at all times) is to busy yourself with an easy physical task, like washing up, vacuuming, ironing or gardening. Based on a Zen principle, this will occupy your lower self; then your higher mind can observe what's going on.

Observing your thought patterns

Choose your task, then decide firmly that you will become the observer, watching the thoughts in your mind.

Allow the thoughts to flow in and out and do not give them any energy; do not react to them either in a positive or in a negative way. When a thought comes in, just observe it quietly, gently. Do not fight any negative thoughts by telling them how horrible they are, as "What you resist will persist" and the thought will "dig its heels in" and want to stay with you even longer. Negative attention will produce more negativity, as like attracts like.

All the thoughts you have are of equal value, be they "good" or "bad". Remember that the so-called " bad" ones, only show you where more love and healing is needed in your life.

Write down your findings. It may take some days or even weeks for tangible patterns to emerge. (Please have patience with yourself. This is such a valuable and important exercise; do not give up on it!)

> *"Since even wild animals can gradually be trained with patience,*
> *the human mind also can gradually be trained step by step."*
> *—His Holiness the Dalai Lama*

As you have observed, and are now aware of, some of the negative thoughts and beliefs you carry around with you, we move on to the next step of making sure that you are truly willing to release and let go of them.

We all crave LOVE and positive attention, and we will go out of our way to get it.

If we cannot "get hold of love" in a natural way, we will find other ways (this process happens mostly in the subconscious), creating some kind of problem in order to get the attention and love we so much crave.

Subconsciously, we create and hold onto negative patterns of behaviour, be they mental, emotional or physical, because we receive a "pay-off" from them. The "pay-off" involves bartering our self-created misery for a kernel of attention or an ounce of love.

A "pay off" is a mental or emotional attachment that is holding our negative patterns of over/under-eating, taking drugs, drinking too much alcohol, excessive exercise and sex or whatever, in place. This attachment is fuelled by the fear of giving it up, as whatever it is we are currently trying to give up in our lives involves change, and the notion of change induces fear of the unknown. We worry that when the familiar structures and behaviour patterns are gone, we will not be able to cope, with this new, empty state of being.

There is only one way and one substance to fill the void, your love for yourself and the light of your father/mother God!

You might like to repeat "Releasing attachments to the past and future affirmations" from Part 2: God Matters at this point. Now we will take this process a step further and move into letting go of the "pay offs".

Some of your personal pay-offs may have come up already in the work we have done, but here are some possible examples for you.

(Since this book has your body-shape as its main focus, we will concentrate on this area most. However the same principle applies for all other areas of your life.)

LETTING GO OF "PAY-OFFS EXERCISE"

Here are some of the "pay offs" or bartering tools you might be using:

"If I stay in this pattern of behaviour:

I can prove to you that I am not lovable.

I can prove to you that I don't deserve to be loved.

I can carry on stopping people from loving me.

I can demonstrate to you how much I need you.

I can demonstrate to you how poor I am.

I can carry on telling you how many problems I have.

I can carry on telling you how difficult my life is.

I can carry on complaining about my life.

I can always find another reason to fail.

I can carry on punishing myself.

I can carry on feeling guilty and miserable.

I can prove that I cannot and never will be perfect."

Please think of your specific pay-off patterns and make a list.

Next, you can use the power of affirmations to programme your mind with the positive opposites of the negative pay-offs on your list.

The following examples from the list above will show you how to do this.

I, _(your name)____, am lovable because I AM.

I,_____, deserve to be loved, no matter what I do or how I perform.

I,_____, allow people to love me the best way they are able to.

I, _____ ,am capable of fulfilling my own needs effortlessly.

I, _____ , am naturally wealthy in body, mind, emotions and spirit.

I, _____ , am perfectly capable of coping with my problems.

I, _____ , am able to overcome the difficulties in my life with ease.

I, _____ , feel no more need to complain.

I, _____ , am blessed with success in all my endeavours.

I, _____ , love and appreciate my efforts.

I, _____ , am free of guilt, which has been projected on to me.

I, _____ , am a perfect child of God.

Keep on writing those positive affirmations, until they actually feel true to you.

You will succeed!

To make sure that you release your negative thoughts and beliefs completely, I will now take you through a series of visualisation. These will employ the creative power of your mind, together with the light and love of God, to clear your mind of all negativity and bring you closer to your chosen goal.

To assure your success, please read through the following instructions before beginning the visualisations.

Energy work made easy

Before you start with the visualisations or any other energy work please make sure that you

- have at least 30 minutes of undisturbed time to yourself

- invite an angel to bless your meditation space

- are comfortable.

While doing these energy processes, you may sit in the lotus position or in a chair, or if you feel more comfortable you may lie down. I would advise you to sit upright, with your spine straight; it will help you to keep your attention focused on the task ahead.

If sitting in a chair, rest your hands in an open position on your lap, with your feet planted firmly on the ground.

You might want to have a blanket ready in case you feel chilly during the exercise.

It is a good idea to start keeping a journal, in which you record your observations, findings and general progress.

This journal will not only provide a useful and interesting record for the future, but will also show you how far you have come and how well you have done!

Follow the sequence outlined in Part 3 Light connections: the five step process

1) **Aligning with God's divine will and purpose**

2) **Aligning with the earth energies – grounding**

3) **Aligning with the heavens attunement**

4) **Closing down the chakras and protecting your auric field**

5) **Giving thanks**

Mind clearing processes

Here are three different approaches that will greatly help to clear your mind of negative thought forms:

MIND CLEARING EXERCISE NUMBER 1: THE GOLDEN BUBBLE

Make sure that you sit comfortably and that the phone is off the hook.

Now take three deep breaths.

As you breathe in, think "I am aligning myself with God's divine will" and on the out-breath think "I am releasing and letting go of all that is not love".

As you do this you will feel a wave of relaxation wash over you.

Your feet will start to feel heavy…

Your shoulders will drop…

Your jaw and neck muscles will relax…

On the next in-breath, start to grow golden roots from the soles of your feet.

As you breathe out, release and let go.

Let the golden roots travel through the layers of the earth until you arrive at a depth where you feel comfortably grounded.

Now become aware of a force field of golden light, which is all around you.

Take a deep breath in and allow this energy to flow into the top of your head, your crown chakra, and from there to the next chakra, your third eye.

Place your awareness into your third eye and observe your thoughts for a while.

You might perceive your thoughts as an inner knowing, as flashes of energy, or you might see them as pictures; some people can even taste negative thought-forms.

When the next negative thought-form comes in, imagine the golden light, which is the Christ-healing light, forming a bubble around it and completely sealing it up tight.

Take a deep breath in and release the bubble, which you can now see sailing out of your third eye chakra and floating up into the sky.

As you look up into the sky, you become aware of a group of healing angels with butterfly nets. The healing angels catch the golden bubble filled with your negative thought form and fly off with it to source, where it will be transmuted into light.

Now repeat the process with the next negative thought form… and so on.

Then close down your chakras.

Start by visualising your chakras as wooden gates and imagine the gates to be made of solid oak wood, with sturdy locks complete with ornate golden keys.

When you are ready, firmly shut the first gate – the crown chakra – turning the golden key in the lock.

Repeat the same closing process all the way down. From the crown chakra move to the third eye chakra, then the throat chakra, the heart chakra, the solar plexus chakra, the sacral chakra and finally close the base chakra. When you are ready, draw up your golden roots, leaving them just a few inches deep in the ground.

Now imagine a huge bubble of golden Christ-light in front of you.

You can make its colour as light and bright as you like and its consistency as light or dense as you like. The bubble could look very airy, or almost liquid if you feel you need stronger protection. It can be any size, so long as you can walk into it.

You don't need to think about this, your higher mind with the help of God and the healing angels will produce the perfect bubble for you.

Take a step forward and walk right into it.

You are now perfectly protected and the golden light will carry on nourishing you during the rest of your day.

Give thanks to God and to the healing angels for their assistance.

Use the following exercise, when you have a "heavy mind", with negative thoughts weighing you down.

MIND CLEARING EXERCISE NUMBER 2: THE GLASS TUBE

Make sure that you are comfortable and your phone is turned off.

Take a deep breath, aligning your self with God's will on the in-breath and releasing all negativity on the out-breath.

Become aware of God's love and light all around you.

As you carry on breathing you become more and more relaxed.

Your legs become heavier and heavier…

Your arms flop into your lap…

Your stomach area relaxes…

Your shoulders drop…

Now, on the next in-breath visualise golden roots from the soles of your feet, growing into the ground.

Your golden roots are growing down and down, through the layers of the earth, where they find a large, solid rock and wrap themselves around it.

Now become aware of a bright, white energy surrounding you.

This white energy feels light and crisp.

Take a deep breath in and visualise this bright white energy flowing into your crown chakra filling it with light.

On the next in-breath, the bright white light flows from the crown chakra into your third eye chakra, flooding it with light.

(If at this point you feel a slight headache coming on, do not worry. This is a psychic headache due to the clearing you are doing and will soon pass. If it intensifies, stop the exercise immediately and re-ground yourself, before you come out of it.)

Next imagine a glass tube, attached to your brow, over your third eye chakra.

At the end of the tube you see a couple of healing angels hovering in mid-air, holding a golden bucket under the end of the tube.

Now take a deep breath in and tell your mind to expel all negative, disruptive thoughts through this tube.

You watch in amazement as a vast variety of negative thoughts leave your mind.

You might see objects or colours travelling through the tube or you might just know intuitively what you are releasing.

When the golden bucket is full, the healing angels take it back to source, where the negative energy gets transmuted into light.

Carry on filling up the golden bucket as long as necessary.

When you are finished, start to close down your chakras.

Imagine your chakras to be solid, heavy silver trap doors, held open by strong, sturdy silver chains.

See yourself grabbing hold of the chains and feel the cool energy of the metal and the texture of the silver. Get a sense of how strong the chains are.

In your own time, when you are ready, release the silver chains and see and feel each silver trapdoor shut with a hefty clank.

Start at the crown chakra and work your way down through the rest of the chakras, ending at the base chakra.

With the chakras firmly closed, you are now ready to unwrap your roots from the rock and slowly bring them up through the layers of the earth.

Leave them in just a few inches deep for extra grounding during the rest the day.

Meanwhile your guardian angel is in attendance to hand you your cloak of protection.

The cloak is made from heavy, midnight-blue velvet with a silver satin lining. It is floor length, with full sleeves, a large hood and diamond clasps, which, when you put the cloak on, are situated exactly over your chakras.

The cloak fits you perfectly, covering and protecting you from top to toe.

Give thanks to God, your guardian angel and the healing angels for their assistance.

The following exercise is particularly helpful, if you have a lot going on in your life and you are feeling stressed, with a brain buzzing with a trillion thoughts and you find it difficult to focus and concentrate on one thing at the time.

MIND CLEARING EXERCISE NUMBER 3: THE ALPHABET

Make sure that you are comfortable and your phone is switched off.

Take a deep breath, aligning your self with the divine will of God on the in-breath

and then releasing all that is not love on the out-breath.

Repeat three times.

As you do this, you slowly become aware that a beautiful, soothing energy field of love and light is surrounding you.

With every breath you take, your body becomes more relaxed.

First your feet begin to feel heavy and the soles of your feet feel as though they are sinking into the ground.

Then the rest of you relaxes, bit by bit…

Your neck…

Your shoulders…

Your body…

Your legs…

With another deep breath you feel much more relaxed…

As you breathe in, imagine golden roots growing from the soles of your feet into mother earth.

The roots grow through the layers of the earth until they stop at a fossilised tree trunk at the core of the earth.

Your roots now firmly wrap themselves around the tree trunk and you are very well grounded indeed.

Next, you become aware of a beam of lemon-yellow light above your head.

This energy is a bright, sparkling light yellow and as you take a breath in you feel this energy entering the top of you head, your crown chakra.

It quickly fills your whole skull with bright yellow light.

Once this is done, put your awareness on your thought patterns.

As you do this you observe millions of letters of the alphabet, swirling around in your brain, all fighting for attention.

They behave like a swarm of bees and you cannot make head nor tail of what your thoughts actually are trying to tell you.

You now decide that there is only one way forward, and that is to eliminate this alphabet soup!

You take another deep breath in and allow the yellow light to fill all the nooks and crannies of your brain.

The bright, sparkling light permeates every letter of the alphabet, and as it does so, the energy is neutralised and you are left with a feeling of calm.

With every breath you take, more and more yellow energy comes in, transmuting more and more of your negative thoughts, letter by letter, word by word, into pure light.

Soon the buzzing in your head stops and you are left with a wonderful feeling of stillness.

Allow this feeling to trickle through the rest of your chakras, all the way down to your feet.

Dwell in the energy of calm and stillness for as long as you wish.

When you have done so, you are ready to close down your chakras.

Starting with the crown chakra, imagine that all your chakras are like open lotus flowers.

Try to get a sense of this magnificent sacred flower and visualise its beautiful, elegant petals.

When you are ready, see the petals slowly closing down until the lotus resembles a bud.

Do the same all the way down to your base chakra.

With your chakras safely closed, you are now ready to unwrap your golden roots from the fossilised tree trunk and bring them up through the layers of the earth, back into the soles of your feet.

It is advisable to leave them just a few inches in the earth, to give you a little extra grounding during the day.

Now it's time to protect yourself.

Visualise a cosy, bright sky-blue, downy sleeping bag with a strong metallic zip.

When you are ready, climb into the sleeping bag and zip up.

As soon as you have done that, you feel safe and cosy, surrounded by the protective blue energy of the sleeping bag.

Give thanks to God, mother earth and the beings of light, which are always in attendance even if you are not aware of it.

> **"He who knows another is wise.**
> **He who knows himself is enlightened."**
> **—Lao Tzu**

Part 5:
Emotional matters

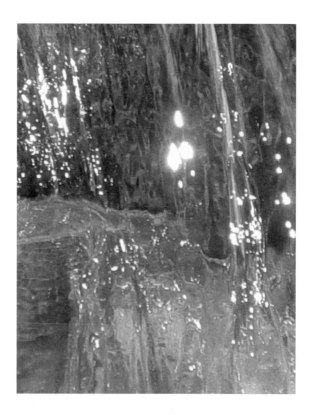

"Your joy is your sorrow unmasked.
And the self-same well from which your laughter rises
was oftentimes filled with your tears.
And how else can it be?"
— *Kahlil Gibran, The Prophet*

The nature of emotions

The dictionary defines emotions as "A strong feeling, such as anger, joy or sadness; an instinctive, intuitive feeling rather than reasoning or knowledge."

Our emotions affect the way we see and experience life. This is perfectly highlighted by the following experiment: A group of trainee police officers were shown a video of a crime. When they were interviewed individually afterwards, it turned out that, although they'd all seen the same video, each police officer gave a slightly different account of the events that they had witnessed on screen.

We can't help but "colour" what we're witnessing with our emotional reaction to it, which immediately makes our observations subjective.

If what we witness is of a non-emotive nature, like someone walking into a supermarket, the chances are that we'll give an accurate account of the event.

If we witness the same person walking into the supermarket and getting mugged, our emotions are aroused and our account of the actual happening will be clouded by our reaction. Furthermore, if a person who's previously been mugged themselves is watching this scene, their emotional reaction to the event will be much stronger than that of a person who'd never experienced a mugging.

Our feelings are coloured by our previous mental, emotional, physical and spiritual experiences, coupled with the mood we are in at the moment.

If we are in a good mood, in a positive emotional state when something bad happens, we are much more able to deal with it in a positive manner.

If we are already in a bad mood, in a negative emotional state, the same event will throw us much more easily.

Very simply put, the process looks like this:

Good mood (such as feeling confident) – we feel happy – resulting in joyful positive behaviour.

Bad mood (such as feeling fear) – we feel unhappy – resulting in destructive negative behaviour.

Many wonderful things may have already happened to us in this lifetime; however, we would not have been able to fully appreciate them if we were in a negative emotional state when they took place.

At other times, just because we were in a positive emotional state, something pleasant but minor may have uplifted and pleased us immensely.

The key to our future happiness, starting from now, lies in controlling and monitoring our emotional states, releasing the old negative ones, coupled with allowing the light and love of God to flow freely into our life.

"And could you keep your heart in wonder at the daily miracles of your life,
your pain would not seem less wondrous than your joy."
—Kahlil Gibran, The Prophet

The origin of emotions

To gain some control over our emotions we need to have a look at where they originate.

To all intents and purposes, it seems that the emotions we feel at any given time are generated from outside of ourselves, being the result of an event which happens to us.

Something happens on the outside and our emotional state immediately changes on the inside.

However, this is not the complete picture.

Most of our emotional responses are triggered by the way the mind perceives or "represents" our reality. The sounds, pictures and dialogues which go on in our mind create for each of us a "unique reality", which may well not be the reality of the next person you meet.

The ongoing processes of the mind, thought by thought, second by second, trigger off a host of emotional responses and are responsible for the greater part of our feelings.

If we liken the mind to a huge computer, the negative thought and belief patterns, which are stored in this vast machinery and still active in the subconscious, will greatly influence the present reality the mind is creating.

It follows that if we are able to clear the negative memories from the subconscious, the mind stands a much better chance of creating a pleasant reality in the here and now.

> *"Know thyself, and thou shalt know the universe."*
> *—Socrates*

The body also plays a part by influencing and storing feelings.

When we have a fright the body automatically clicks into a "flight or fight" reaction and strong negative emotions are aroused. On the other hand, when we relax at yoga class after a long, stressful day, calm, positive emotions are experienced.

This demonstrates that we can induce a positive emotional state by changing the way we use our bodies, since changes in your breathing, posture, muscle tension and facial expression have a direct effect on how we feel and behave.

Some negative emotions, such as the fear felt at the point of experiencing an accident, become literally locked into the muscle fibres of the physical body.

Such locked in emotions inhibit the body from functioning perfectly and result in unexplainable aches and pains.

Such events also have an adverse effect on the mind, which stores the negative memory of an accident away in the subconscious, resulting in possible irrational fears.

By gentle physical manipulation, such as Osteopathy, the old emotional memories can be released from the body, which in turn helps to clear them from the subconscious mind and restore health.

Our state of mind + the physiological state of our body + outside influences produce our feelings.

Here are some guidelines for achieving and maintaining good emotional health:

- *Clear past negative experiences and old negative beliefs and thought patterns from the subconscious mind.*

- *Clear the mind of present negative beliefs, thought-patterns and projections.*

- *Shield ourselves from unnecessary negativity.*

- *Think positively.*

- *Release stuck emotions from the physical body.*

- *Make sure that we are in the best possible physical health.*

- *Attend regular relaxation classes or spend time in nature.*

The function of emotions

Our emotions act as messengers. Their main function is to demand that we pay attention to something that is happening to us right now.

They are signals pointing out what we are experiencing in the present moment.

The more urgent the message the emotions seek to deliver, the stronger the signal, the stronger the feelings we experience.

If we don't listen to our emotions and allow ourselves to express them in some way, their suppression may result in a variety of diseases.

For instance, suppressing the emotion of anger for a prolonged period of time may lead to a depressive state.

The heart is the seat of the emotions and also the seat of the soul.

Emotions are the language of the soul, its attempt at impressing its wisdom upon us.

Sadly, this fact has been widely ignored by western civilisation until fairly recently.

The truth is that we each possess a highly evolved emotional intelligence, of which we are often not entirely aware.

Our hearts contain true wisdom, a gift from the Creator father/mother God, which is there for our taking. Our emotions will speak to us if we only let them.

We can start right now by listening within and paying attention to our soul's messages.

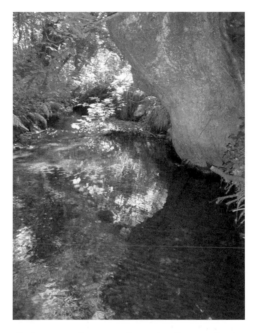

"The head does not hear unless the heart desires to listen."
— author unknown

The purpose of the following visualisation is to allow the emotions you are currently feeling to speak to you, so that you can become clear about their purpose.

You need to approach this visualisation with positive intent, expecting that your emotions will definitely cooperate and share their wisdom with you.

Get the most from this exercise by employing an attitude of love and respect for your emotional body and heart chakra. Endeavour to be loving and grateful for what you are about to receive, thus evoking the divine law of grace in your favour.

ACCESSING YOUR EMOTIONS VISUALISATION

Please allow at least 30 minutes for this exercise and make sure that you are undisturbed during that time.

Make sure, that you are comfortable and your phone is turned off.

When you are ready, take a deep breath in.

As you breathe in, mentally align yourself with God's divine will and purpose.

As you breathe out, release and let go of anything which is not love.

With every breath you take, you become more and more aware of a force field of loving energy surrounding you.

You now start to relax…

Allow your legs and arms to become heavy…

Allow your feet to become heavy….

Allow your shoulders to drop…

Allow your neck and jaw muscles to relax…

Now start to grow golden roots from the soles of your feet, down through the layers of the earth.

When you roots have reached a level you feel comfortable with, allow them to stay there, to ground you for the rest of the exercise. Become aware of a rose-pink vibration surrounding you.

This is a gentle energy which feels like light fluffy pink feathers filling your aura.

You feel safe and protected as if you were ensconced in a heavenly four-poster bed.

Now place one hand over your heart and the other hand on top of it.

Sit back and allow yourself to feel the energy of your heart chakra.

After a little while, you'll sense that you've made a connection with an emotion:

Acknowledge this emotion by saying "Thank you for showing me what I need to learn about myself."

Next try to sense what this particular emotion feels like…

Allow yourself to go with the feeling…

Now speak directly to the emotion you have accessed and ask it where it originates and what it would like to teach you.

Give yourself time to listen.

The answer might come in the form of inspirations, pictures or feelings.

Thank your emotion for coming into your conscious awareness.

When you are ready, start to close down your chakras.

Imagine that your chakras are like pink roses.

Try to visualise these roses in their full splendour with large, sweetly scented petals.

Now see the petals slowly closing until they form a firm bud.

Start with your crown chakra and end with your base chakra.

When you have done this, draw your golden roots up through the layers of the earth, leaving them in the ground just a few inches deep to provide extra grounding during the rest of your day.

Your guardian angel is now ready to hand you a cloak of protection.

This magnificent floor-length cloak is fashioned from rose-pink velvet, lined with bright blue satin, with long sleeves and a large hood.

You put it on and it fits you perfectly.

You feel loved by your guardian angel and are well protected for the remainder of your day.

Give thanks to God and your guardian angel for the love and light you have received.

Another way to discover the valuable gifts hidden within your emotions is to write a letter just to, and then from, your heart. In the first letter you thank your heart and ask it to help you. In the second letter you allow your heart, which has a supreme intelligence of its own, to speak to you.

LETTER FROM YOUR HEART EXERCISE

Make sure that you are undisturbed for at least 30 minutes or so.

Take your phone off the hook and lock your front door.

Make sure you sit in a comfortable position.

Get pen and paper ready.

Be still for a little while.

Take a gentle breath in and release and let go on the out-breath.

Repeat three times, releasing and letting go in the process.

Now write at the top of the page:

To the heart of _____(your name)_____

> Dear heart of mine,
>
> First I would like to thank you for being there for me and working so hard on my behalf. I am eternally grateful for all you do for me on a daily basis and apologize for ignoring the signals you have been sending me. I also would like to say a very big sorry for having abused your services and ask you to forgive me for what I have done.
>
> I am asking you to be so kind as to write a letter to me today, since at present I am not sure of the meaning of the emotions I am experiencing.
>
> I am unable to see the gift that is there for me to use and learn from.
>
> Would you please shed some light on this issue?
>
> With lots of love and light
>
> Yours truly

_____

Enter your signature

Now, without thinking, swiftly start to write down the answer that is coming straight from your heart:

> My dearest (your name)
>
> With lots of love and many blessings
>
> From your loving heart

When you have received an answer thank your heart profoundly for communicating with you so readily.

You can repeat this exercise as often as needed; it will always work and is a wonderful tool, helping you to find the hidden gifts God has bestowed on you.

"The cave you fear to enter holds the treasure you seek."
—Joseph Campbell

The source of unresolved negative emotions

Most of our deep-seated, unresolved negative emotions are old emotions, stemming from our formative years, and will have been caused by some kind of mental, emotional or physical abuse earlier in our lives.

More often than not, we are unable to associate our present feelings with past experiences, as at times they have been so painful that the mind, by way of protecting us, has pushed the original experiences into the subconscious. This is where they still are today in a kind of slumber, but dangerously festering away and with the slightest external stimulation they come out to play, mostly causing havoc in the process.

Most of us have experienced the behaviour of friends or family who seemingly are all "sweetness and light" and then, at the smallest disturbance in their daily routine, explode and undergo a complete personality change – from light into dark in twenty seconds, which can be a frightening experience for anyone involved, especially a child.

Fear, hate, resentment and bitterness are the main negative emotions humankind carries around, leading to struggle and strife both within families and world at large.

As long as these feelings are present within our auric field, they will create blockages in our chakras, which in turn will have a negative effect on our bodies and a negative influence on our lives as a whole.

A perfect body shape and general well-being can only be achieved when these emotions have been pinpointed and released once and for all.

Let us start by looking at the most crippling of all emotions – fear.

We all live with fear in our lives and mostly experience it on a daily basis.

Fear seems to be walking with us hand in hand through life.

Why is that so?

As all experiences are multi-layered, looking at it from the highest level, fear would imply a lack of trust in God.

For if we had true faith and trust in God, our surrender to Him would be absolute and therefore we would not have the slightest doubt that God would take care of us, as we would trust him completely, there would be no need to worry.

We would truly rest in God, like a babe in His arms.

However, this principle will only work when we have learned to believe and trust that God will look after us and care for us, and again, what holds us back from this belief? It's fear, the fear of being let down if we actually do trust and surrender all to God. Our negative conditioning is telling us not to trust anyone, because we've been harmed and disappointed before.

We are still modelling our concept of God on a parent and also perceiving Him as an agency outside of ourselves.

As our parents will most likely have (non-deliberately) mistreated us in some way or another, our visions and expectations of God are less than favourable and we certainly wouldn't be inclined to put faith in Him. Why should we when we could not trust our parents or guardians? What we need to realise is that our parents, guardians or anyone else who has influenced our lives significantly in a negative manner did the very best they could, with the level of awareness that was available to them at the time.

They could not have done it any better or differently; otherwise they would have done so. This is a very important fact to take on board, accept and internalise.

It requires a lot of sitting down and thinking about our parents' and guardians' lives and what negatively influenced them. Usually, we'll unearth a lack of love in their formative years and realise that their emotional shortcomings have been passed on to us and that if we don't heal our own emotional deficiencies, we'll pass those unresolved emotions on to our children in turn.

Whatever our fears might be, those fears need to be recognised and released in some way.

Let us explore different ways of achieving this by applying a variety of approaches, which will enable you to choose the ones that suit you best.

"Do the thing you fear,
and the death of fear is certain."
—Ralph Waldo Emerson

Letting go of fear

To be able to "move through" and release our fears, we must first allow ourselves to acknowledge them. If we stay in denial of them, they will remain our constant companions throughout our lives, throwing a spanner into the works whenever possible.

Set aside at least half an hour of your time for this exercise.

Make sure your phone is turned off and that you are comfortable.

RELEASING YOUR FEARS VISUALISATION

Question yourself: What is the fear that has the greatest hold on me and most influences my life?

Ask God, the healing angels, the beings of light and your guardian angel for help, and evoke the law of grace by being truly grateful for what you are about to receive.

Breathe in love and light, release and let go on the out-breath.

Ask to be aligned with God's divine will and your highest purpose.

Take a deep breath in and allow your body to relax on the out breath.

Starting with your feet and working up, keep releasing and letting go of any tensions you may hold in your muscles.

Relax your feet…

Relax your legs…

Relax your torso…

Carry on releasing and letting go of all tensions, all the way up to the top of your head.

When you are ready, grow strong golden roots from the soles of your feet, down through the layers of the earth, all the way into mid-earth, where you find a huge, solid rock.

Now allow your golden roots to wrap themselves around this rock.

Meanwhile you become aware of an orange light surrounding you.

This light has a beautiful glow to it and feels both strong and soothing.

Take a deep breath in and allow this light to flow into the top of your head, through your crown chakra.

Allow the orange light to fill your crown chakra.

Now let the orange light flow from your crown into your third eye chakra, filling it with its soothing energy.

From there the orange energy flows into your throat chakra, down to your heart chakra and finally into your solar plexus chakra, the area just above your belly button.

Allow your entire solar plexus centre, the seat of your fears and anxieties to be filled with this orange light.

When this has been achieved, put your left hand on your solar plexus and then place your right hand on top of it.

Now allow yourself to feel the fear that is presenting itself.

You will most likely experience a variety of physical sensations, such as a slight stomach-ache and minor feelings of sickness.

Keep on breathing in the orange light, which will help to alleviate those symptoms.

When you feel you have connected with your fear, visualise yourself sitting in your own private cinema.

Now sit back in your cinema chair and grab the remote control.

You are aware that your fear is about to be uncovered, enabling you to face it once and for all.

Take another deep breath of orange light and in your own time press the start button on the remote control and ask for the origin of your fear to show up on screen.

To your amazement a scene from your life flashes up immediately, in full colour and with sound accompanying it.

Stay focused on your fear and keep on breathing in the orange light.

Now using your remote control, fade the colour out of the scene in front of you, until the movie you are viewing is entirely in black and white.

Observe how the fear is starting to loose its grip on you.

Take another deep breath of the beautiful, soothing orange light.

Release and let go on the out-breath.

Next press the zoom button and shrink the scene until there is only a tiny dot left on the screen.

As you watch, even the dot disappears.

Your fear has been extinguished.

Turn off your remote control and return your awareness to your hands.

You are able to sense that the area around your solar plexus feels a lot calmer now.

Take another deep breath of orange light, let it refill your solar plexus and then allow it to flow from there into your sacral chakra and then into your base chakra, ending in the minor chakras of the soles of your feet.

Your fear has gone and you feel relieved and relaxed at the same time!

When you are ready, start to close down your chakras.

Visualise them as heavy silver trap doors, held open by sturdy silver chains.

You are impressed by how strong they are and how sturdy their construction is.

Get hold of the silver chains and starting with the crown chakra, see and feel the trapdoor shut firmly with a clang.

Repeat all the way down to your base chakra.

In your own good time extract your golden roots from the rock and slowly bring them up through the layers of mother earth, leaving them a few inches deep in the soil to give you some extra grounding during the rest of your day.

Now imagine a large electric-blue downy sleeping bag, with a strong zip in front of you.

Climb into it and zip it up.

You are now nicely protected by the strong electric blue energy surrounding you.

Give thanks for all the heavenly support you've received.

As we've had a look at fears in general, let's now become more specific about those relating to body-shape.

Ask yourself the following question: what are the fears that are holding you back from achieving your perfect body-shape?

Two of the most common fears connected with the subject are:

1. **the fear of failing to achieve your perfect body-shape**
2. **the fear of succeeding in achieving your perfect body-shape**

First on the list is the fear of failure of achieving your perfect body-shape.

To start with, please allow yourself to remember when you were first made to feel that you were a failure.

Was it perhaps in very early childhood when we could not perform certain tasks, such as holding a fork or doing up shoelaces?

(As we now know potty training difficulties may lead to fears of failure in later life.)

Or was it in your junior school days when you could not make the grades or did not perform well on sports day?

Did your father, mother or guardian tell you that you were "good for nothing" as a person?

Did a friend tell you that you were never going to meet the boy/girl of your dreams, because you were a failure?

The following exercise will release this negative conditioning of failure.

CHANGING FAILURES INTO SUCCESSES VISUALISATION

Make sure you have about 30 minutes of undisturbed time available.

Have pen and paper to hand.

Ask for help from God and the beings of light and give thanks for the support you are about to receive.

Make a list of events where you were deemed to be a failure.

Now make sure that you are comfortable.

Take a few gentle breaths and relax.

Align yourself with God's divine will, plan and purpose.

Relax, release and let go of all tensions in your body.

Feel that you are surrounded by a force field of love and light.

Grow your golden roots through the layers of the earth until you feel well grounded.

Feel a rose-coloured energy enveloping you.

Take a deep breath and allow the rose-coloured energy to wash right through all your chakras and fill all the layers of your auric field.

You are now enveloped in a wonderful rose-coloured cocoon.

Take a deep breath and allow the rose coloured energy to flow into the top of your head and from there all the way into your heart chakra and finally into your solar plexus area.

Now look at the first item on your list.

This will most likely be your most vivid memory. Attempt to relive the event in your mind, making the scenes as vivid as you can.

See the negative memory like a film playing on the screen of your third eye.

Try to remember the time of day, any sounds, colours or smells which were present.

When it's over, play an alternative positive version of the event on your inner screen.

Try to make this version bright and colourful.

In this updated version you are a brilliant success and you are very happy with your achievements.

See yourself smiling and happy and others congratulating you on your fantastic accomplishment.

Repeat this process all the way through your list, one by one reprogramming your mind and emotions from failure to success.

When you have finished become aware again of the rose-coloured energy and let it flow from your solar plexus all the way into the soles of your feet.

When you have done so, close down your chakras.

See them as wooden gates that have sturdy locks with golden keys in them.

One by one, starting at the crown chakra you shut the wooden gate behind you, turning the key in the lock, before you move on to the next one.

When you have done so, begin to draw your golden roots back into the soles of your feet, just leaving them in a few inches deep, enough to provide some grounding for the rest of the day.

Finally imagine a huge bubble of golden light in front of you.

When you are ready, step forward and right into the golden bubble.

This energy that is the golden healing light closes in around you and you are perfectly safe and protected.

Give thanks for all the help you have received.

As you delete memory after negative memory from your mind, your fear of failure will diminish and finally disappear.

You may, most likely, have to go through this exercise several times before all traces of your fear of failure have been extinguished.

Now to the second item on the list: the fear of actually achieving your perfect body shape.

It does not seem logical at first, but fear of success is nearly as widespread as fear of failure and can often share common roots.

If you succeed in your achievements, it can mean giving up a whole list of pay-offs, as we've discussed earlier.

You might subconsciously hang on to your weight problems because they give you some sort of stability and personal identity.

Here, to jog your memory, are some examples to get you started compiling your own list:

Examples:

- I am afraid of being too perfect, my friends would be jealous of me.
- I am afraid of being too beautiful and getting too much attention.
- I am afraid of "having it all" and then nobody would like me.
- I am afraid of being too powerful.
- I am afraid that people would have high expectations of me.
- I am afraid that I could not handle all this change.

In the next exercise you will write up your own list, leaving some spaces between the lines. You will need to do some soul searching. It will be worth it in the end.

RELEASING YOUR FEARS OF SUCCESS AFFIRMATIONS

Write down the reason for your fear of success and then compose three positive affirmations in the next few lines.

Example:

I _____ fear achieving my perfect body shape because I am afraid that I could not handle all this change _____

Positive affirmations: I am perfectly capable of handling the changes in my life.

I can change whenever I want to.

I find it easy to change.

Try to make your list as comprehensive as possible.

Please read your positive affirmations out loud nine times each and repeat until you start to feel an energy shift.

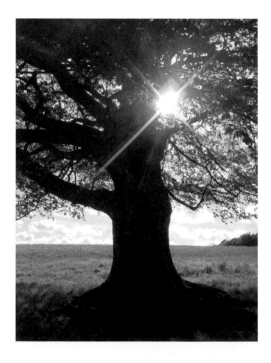

*"Love is the most universal, the most tremendous
and the most mysterious of the cosmic forces."*
—Pierre Teilhard de Chardin

❀   ❀   ❀

THE HATE, SHAME AND BLAME GAME

Hate is another strong, destructive emotion brought on by a lack of love for ourselves or a lack of love from others.

The emotion of hate is often closely linked to shame, giving rise, in many instances to blame.

As in essence the self is all there is and the world around us reflects what's going on inside us, let's start with the emotion of self-hate.

The hate we have for another is exactly the same amount of hate we have for ourselves. We are projecting our inner world of hate, born from lack of love for ourselves, on to the outer world.

Feelings of self-hate are intrinsically linked with feelings of shame. If there are strong emotions of hate, shame is never far away. Mixed in with these destructive emotions is another one, guilt. Guilt can only arise if it's projected on to us by an outside agency. If you were the only person on this planet going along doing your own thing, no matter how stupid or dangerous your behaviour or acts were, would you ever feel guilty about it? No.

We cannot feel guilty all by ourselves; there needs to be someone making us feel guilty, and this is what someone will do if they have their own agenda at heart.

When dealing with guilt, we can remind ourselves of this truth: when we feel guilty we are being emotionally blackmailed. No matter what we've done or not done, according to this outside force, we need to acknowledge that we did the best we could.

We did the best under the circumstances, with the awareness and opportunities available to us at the time. If we could have, we would have done it better or differently.

Hate is a heavy emotion, which sits like huge blobs in the auric field, creating massive energy blocks in the chakras. Retained self-hate is probably the primary cause of eating disorders. We either overeat to dull the emotional pain of self-hate or we starve ourselves in order to punish ourselves for our feelings, often adding to our shame and guilt along the way.

The most intense feelings of hate are generally reserved for family members or close friends and are always linked to having experienced some kind of abuse at their hands, be it mental, emotional, physical or sexual abuse. This too can cause blockages in the auric field.

"Your pain is the breaking of the shell that encloses your understanding."
—Kahlil Gibran, The Prophet

If you feel that you are harbouring issues of hate for others and yourself, complete the following:

Hate, blame and shame exercises:

• *Recognising hate for others*

I, _____ , hate my father because _____

I, _____ , hate my mother because _____

I, _____ , hate my guardians because _____

I, _____ , hate_____ because_____

I, _____ , hate God because _____

• *Acknowledging self-hate*

Please try to dig deep and allow your feelings to come to the surface.

I, _____ , hate myself because _____

I, _____ , hate myself because _____

I, _____ , hate myself because _____

Now let's do the same soul searching exercises to shine some light onto the feelings of shame and guilt.

ACKNOWLEDGING FEELINGS OF SHAME EXERCISE

You'll probably feel self-conscious and maybe even a bit frightened of committing your feelings of shame to paper. Please remember that by writing your feelings down, you have started the process of releasing them.

I, _____ , am ashamed of my feelings because _____

I, _____ , am ashamed of my thoughts because _____

I,_____ , am ashamed of what I would like to say because_____

I,_____ , am ashamed of my body because _____

I,_____ , am ashamed of what I would like to do because_____

I,_____ , am ashamed of what has happened to me because_____

TRACING FEELINGS OF GUILT

As you have now become aware, guilt is a projected emotion; allow yourself to search for the origins of your guilt feelings.

I, _____ , feel guilty about being happy because_____

I, _____ , feel guilty about wanting to be beautiful because_____

I, _____ , feel guilty about my body-shape because _____

I, _____ , feel guilty for wanting to lead my own life because_____

I, _____ , feel guilty about wanting to be loved because _____

"*A traveller I am and a navigator,*
***and every day I discover a new region within my soul.*"**
—*Kahlil Gibran, The Prophet*

And finally try to be as honest as you can with yourself.

Who and what is it you are blaming your misfortunes on?

This is the "blame game", a way of passing the buck, which will lead you round in ever-decreasing circles, never achieving any positive solutions in your life.

All of us have played this game at one time or another and some of us have become so good at it that the game we play seem to be real and become habitual.

The point of the game is this: "If I carry on blaming others for the things which are not working in my life, for instance, trying to achieve my perfect body-shape, I take the focus off what's really going on within me, and project it on to the outside world. This gives me the perfect excuse for staying just the way I am. In this case either too fat or too thin and, in general, not happy with either my body-shape or my life."

WHY I BLAME OTHERS

This is the hour of truth.

Now, please own up and write down your blame routines:

I, _____ , blame my mother for_____

I, _____ , blame my father for _____

I, _____ , blame my friends for_____

I, _____ , blame God for_____

I, _____ , blame the world for_____

If this game is not working out too well, then you might try to play the game of

"I blame myself instead and feel guilty in the bargain".

Allow yourself to have a look at what you are currently blaming yourself for.

Here are some suggestions: your life, the way you look, what you have done or not done etc.

EXERCISE: WHY I BLAME MYSELF

I, _____ , *blame myself for*_____

I, _____ , *blame myself for*_____

I, _____ , *blame myself for*_____

Please carry on writing down all that comes to your mind at this moment.

Forgiveness, the key to healing

We have done some very thorough soul-searching in the last few exercises of this book and confronted many of our fears. As we have pointed the torchlight of our soul at the unloved aspects of our personality and have acknowledged and accepted our findings, no matter how painful and disturbing they might have been, it's now time to wholly and finally release our old fears and any other remaining emotional baggage.

The golden key of forgiveness, a magical tool for transformation, is available to us for this purpose.

The act of forgiveness washes away all residues of bitterness, hate, doubt, fear and resentment. The bright energy of forgiveness sweeps away the dark, murky energies of our stuck emotions and allows the light of our hearts to illuminate the entire self. All stored up negative emotions will simply be melted away and transmuted into light.

Without true forgiveness welling up from within our own beautiful hearts, our journey to self-healing and achieving our perfect body-shape will just be a mental concept which will never be fulfilled.

We have the power to do this and the choice is ours.

Complete forgiveness will take time, for some of us longer than for others, depending on the issues and the amount of love and light in our hearts available to us at present. We need not force the issue; we can take this process slowly, honouring ourselves for every step we take. We can align the ego will with the divine will, hand the process over to God and the healing angels, and trust it to be done!

> *"Where love rules, there is no willpower and where power predominates, there love is lacking.*
> *The one is the shadow of the other."*
> *—C. J. Jung*

Start your journey of forgiveness with these essential, positive affirmations.

As your negative emotions have been in place for a long time, at times even carried through from past lives into this life, you need to make a supreme effort with these affirmations, the light of which will melt away all that is not love.

Please write each affirmation out 90 times. Yes, 90, for a number of reasons.

First, 90 is a completion number; second, your forgiveness process will take time to reach all the levels of your being. The energy of forgiveness needs to deeply penetrate your subconscious mind in order to erase all negativity stored there.

Before you do any of the affirmations please take a deep breath and consciously connect with your higher self, asking for its cooperation with you in releasing all negativity out of your auric field once and for all.

FORGIVENESS AFFIRMATIONS

• *From hate to forgiveness*

I, _____, *completely forgive my father.*

I, _____, *completely forgive my mother.*

I, _____, *completely forgive my guardians.*

I, _____, *completely forgive God.*

• *From self-hate to self-forgiveness*

I, _____, *wholly forgive myself for anything I think I might have thought, said or done wrong.*

I, _____, *wholly forgive myself for not trusting and believing in myself.*

I, _____, *wholly forgive myself for hating myself*

I, _____, *wholly forgive myself for not trusting in God.*

• *From blame to forgiveness*

I, _____, *now forgive my mother for*_____

I, _____, *now forgive my father for*_____

I, _____ , *now forgive my guardians for* _____

I, _____ , *now forgive my friends for* _____

I, _____ , *now forgive God for* _____

I, _____ , *now forgive the world for* _____

The person you are most harsh with is always yourself.

Give yourself a cuddle and forgive yourself.

Apply the divine sticking plaster of self-forgiveness whenever you feel stuck in any way; you'll be surprised how many times self-loathing in one form or another was behind your negative emotions.

• *From self-blame to self-forgiveness*

I, _____ , *forgive myself for overeating/not eating.*

I, _____ , *forgive myself for hating my body.*

I, _____ , *forgive myself for hurting myself/others.*

• *Using the light of forgiveness affirmations*

I, _____ , *love and forgive myself unconditionally.*

I, _____ , *allow the light of forgiveness to shine into every corner of my being.*

I, _____ , *offer the light of forgiveness to others and allow them to love me.*

I, _____ , *allow the light of God to nourish me.*

> **AND SO BE IT.**
> **AND SO BE IT.**
> **AND SO BE IT.**
> **I AM THE I AM.**
> **I AM THE I AM.**
> **I AM THE I AM.**

Give thanks for all the love and divine sustenance you've received.

With every completed affirmation the light of your forgiveness will dissolve another pain and heal another wound.

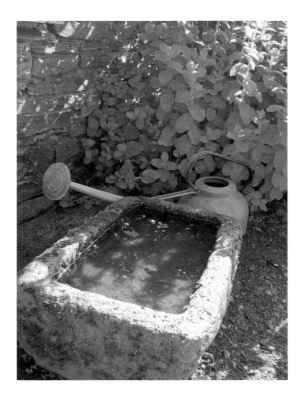

"Do not disregard the accumulation of goodness, saying,
"This will come to nothing".
By the gradual falling of raindrops, a jar is filled."
—The Buddha

The divine seal of blessings

There is just one final act which makes the forgiveness process complete, and that is the act of asking for divine blessings.

This is seemingly a very simple gesture, but I cannot stress the importance of it highly enough, as the divine energy of the blessing acts as a seal of light and will efficiently dissolve the last remaining vestiges of any negativity still present.

A divine blessing humbly evoked by you and administered by God will make your forgiveness process complete. The following blessing affirmations and visualisations demonstrate how to do this.

BLESSING AFFIRMATIONS

I, _____ , *humbly ask for my life to be blessed.*

I, _____ , *humbly ask you God to bless every thought I think.*

I, _____ , *humbly ask you God to bless every word I speak.*

I, _____ , *humbly ask you God to bless all the deeds I perform.*

I, _____ , *humbly ask for my body, mind, emotions and spirit to be blessed.*

I, _____ , *humbly ask for my past, present and future to be blessed.*

I, _____ , *humbly ask for my father to be blessed.*

I, _____ , *humbly ask for my mother to be blessed.*

I, _____ , *humbly ask for my guardians to be blessed.*

I, _____ , *humbly ask for my friends to be blessed.*

I, _____ , *humbly ask for all my soul brothers and soul sisters and mother earth to be blessed.*

Please feel free to add many more blessings to this list.

Work with the following visualisation by picturing the divine light of God's blessings being poured over any person or situation you would like to heal.

BLESSING VISUALISATION

As always, align yourself with the divine will.

Take a deep breath, relax and ground yourself.

Know that you are surrounded by a force field of love and light.

Then imagine the person, animal, place or situation you would like to be blessed appearing on your inner screen.

Make the picture as vivid as possible, adding colour and sound, feeling, smell and taste.

Now, from your heart, ask God to bless the scene you are witnessing.

Immediately you become aware of a beam of golden healing light, entering the top of your head, swiftly filling your crown chakra and then proceeding to flow into your third eye chakra.

There you watch in amazement as everything you see is first bathed in golden light, and then permeated by the golden light.

The image becomes lighter and lighter until finally all negativity is erased.

Carry on with your visualisation, allowing the movie in your mind to run its light-filled course to the end.

When the movie has ended, close down your chakras.

Bring your roots back into the soles of your feet and protect yourself.

Give thanks for the divine blessings you've received.

Cutting cords – releasing negative energy connections

As we are all ONE and connected to each other on the highest levels of existence, we are also connected to each other on all the other levels of our being.

We talk about family ties, for instance, families are held together by a common history and mutual feelings of love and respect for each other.

These ties are of a mental and emotional fabric, made from psychic matter.

As thoughts and feelings are vibrations, when we think about someone or feel any emotions for them, an energy connection is made and if the other person responds, then a tie is formed between both individuals.

For example, when we were born, in the same way that the umbilical cord physically connected us to our mother, we would have had an energy cord running from our solar plexus to our mother's solar plexus. We would also have had other cords with our mother connecting her chakras with ours.

These are the psychic ties, which bind humans together on the mental and emotional levels. However these ties may have a negative mental, emotional or even physical effect.

If the ties between us and another are of a "light nature", that is to say the connection is one of unconditional love, then the ties will act as conduits of love and light and be of a beneficial nature.

Sadly, this is rarely the case. In reality, we are hardly ever able to conduct our affairs, whether they be of the heart, the mind or the body, with unconditional love. Therefore the cords that connect us are mostly held in place by the opposite of love, namely, fear. Any energy connected to us that is not of pure love has the ability to drain our mental, emotional and physical energy reserves by cording into our chakras, even at times, holding back our spiritual development and enjoyment.

To prevent this from happening, we need to learn to love unconditionally. A love without conditions allows the other person to be free to experience what they need to experience in their life.

This is a hard undertaking, as our human love tries to over-protect, to over-nurture and to manipulate and direct the lives of others. Emotionally, we find it extremely hard to give freely, just for the sake and the pure joy and love of giving. We may not be conscious of it, but in the majority of situations we do expect a return for the "good deeds" we've done.

So, a push and pull situation ensues and co-dependency thrives.

This pattern won't change until we can see ourselves for what we are, beings of light, wholly complete in our divinity. We have all the tools we need right there within us to make our lives the success they deserve to be. All the powers of heaven and earth have been gifted to us by our father/mother God. You just need to look for, find, unwrap and use those wonderful gifts. They are ours for the taking.

It is advisable to discover just who it is that is holding you back from achieving what you want and from enjoying the success you so much deserve. This needs to be done with care and respect for all involved.

FINDING NEGATIVE CORDING EXERCISE

Make a list of the usual suspects first, mostly members of your family. Then think about the rest of your friends, work colleagues and acquaintances. Complete your list.

Then, one by one, establish the feeling you get when you are thinking of each individual.

What does it feel like when you visualise each person standing in front of you?

How does their energy affect yours?

Do you feel happy, joyful and uplifted or does your energy drop leaving you feeling sad, angry or depressed by just thinking of them.

What your feelings reveal is clear: anyone who makes you feel low in any way is corded into your energy field in a negative way.

Now underline all the culprits on your list, who depressed your energy.

You'll need this list in the guided meditation that follows.

To begin with just start to cut the cords with one person at a time, especially those you have a lot of issues with. Later on, when you've had some practice and have become familiar with the process, you may cut ties with a whole group of people at once, if appropriate. (An example might be a group of colleagues at work you have problems with.)

The following energy process brings together the elements of cutting the cords: forgiveness, reclaiming your power and sealing the healing process with a blessing.

This is a powerful process and will bring instant results.

Please be aware that the person you are de-cording from will, on a higher level, be aware of this process, which might lead to changes in their behaviour towards you.

React with love towards them and take it as part of the process.

CUTTING THE CORDS VISUALISATION

This is one of the most important visualisations for you to do, so please allow at least 45 minutes of your time.

Make sure not be disturbed by children, pets, doorbells or telephones.

Allow yourself to get comfortable.

Ask God, the healing angels, beings of light and your guardian angels to assist you.

Evoke the law of grace by being grateful for their help and support.

Now take a lovely, deep breath in and mentally align your self with God's divine will, your highest purpose and the highest purpose of anyone else involved in this energy process.

Sense a beautiful loving, kind energy enveloping you.

You feel totally safe and protected, knowing that God and the beings of light are looking after you.

On the next in-breath allow your body to relax.

Starting from your feet, allow all tensions to drain through your foot chakras into the earth.

Move through your whole body, releasing, relaxing and letting go of all tension...

When you are ready, grow strong golden roots from the soles of your feet through the layers of the earth, all the way into the middle of the earth, where your roots wrap themselves around a sturdy, ancient fossilised tree trunk.

Now you become aware of a sparkling blue light surrounding you.

This is the special healing light of Archangel Michael who has come to aid you in your energy process.

Take a deep breath in and allow this crisp, bright blue light to enter your crown chakra and wash all the way through your energy centres, all the way down to your base chakra.

As you breathe out, release and let go of all that is not love.

The more you focus on the sparkling blue light the stronger it becomes, clearing, cleansing and purifying your chakras and your auric field.

When you feel that you've had a thorough cleansing, visualise yourself sitting on an ornate chair in a temple of light.

The temple is built from gleaming white marble lavishly decorated with magical crystals and beautiful flowers.

You seem to hear fluttering noises and as you look up you see a legion of healing cherubs floating beneath the ceiling.

At this instant you become aware that Archangel Michael is standing to the right of your chair.

He is holding a giant blue sword in his hands; this is the sword of truth.

Archangel Michael now welcomes you and explains that this is the sword he will use to cut all the unhealthy cords connecting you to other people.

He tells you that only the negative aspects of the energy connection will be cut and that the unconditional love link will remain intact.

As unconditional love is light, those cords are all but invisible and can just be felt very lightly.

You are happy with his explanation and now find another chair being put in front of you by the healing angels.

Now, sitting in your chair, ask your higher self to invite the person you need most to de-cord from to come into the healing temple.

See the healing angels accompanying this person into the temple, leading him/her to the chair opposite you.

If you are not able to visualise, you will instead get a strong sense, a knowing who this person is.

Wait for them to sit down.

You can see the cords, like thick ropes running between your chakras and the chakras of the other person, linking you both together.

Some of the cords will be thicker than others, depending on the strength of the mental, emotional or physical ties between you.

Look into this person's eyes, as the eyes are the windows to the soul, and tell them that you are here to cut the unhealthy attachments between you.

Explain to them that you are doing this from the point of unconditional love and that you want to set yourself, and them, free.

The person opposite you at times might seem to be uncomfortable with this idea, but persevere talking to them about your reasons for doing this. Having said all that needs to be said, ask Archangel Michael to raise his sword.

When you are ready, ask him to cut the ties, which he does with one mighty blow of his blue sword.

The cords fall to the ground, where they shrivel up and disappear.

Now, from you heart, forgive the person for what they have done to you.

Then forgive yourself for any negative part you may have played in the relationship.

Finally reclaim the personal power this person has taken from you; just demand it to be returned to you.

You see the person handing you a ball of light representing the displaced energy and you place it in your solar plexus chakra, the seat of your power.

If you have stolen any power, then it is time to return that too.

When this has been done, ask the healing angels for extra healing and blessings for both of you.

They readily flutter down from the ceiling giving you the healing and the blessings you have asked for.

When this is done, the healing angels accompany the person out of the healing temple.

Thank Archangel Michael for his invaluable services and also give thanks to the healing angels for their support and kindness.

See yourself leaving the healing temple walking back into your own meditation room.

Close down your chakras by imagining them to be heavy silver trap doors, held open by strong, sturdy chains. One by one, let go of the chains, closing all your chakras from the crown to the base chakra.

Now unwrap your golden roots from the fossilised tree trunk, bring them back through the layers of the earth, leaving them in a few inches deep for extra grounding.

This done, your guardian angel steps behind you and hands you a mantle of protection, putting it over your shoulders.

The mantle is made from smooth, thick purple velvet and lined with a silver satin lining.

It fits perfectly, covering you from top to toe in its protective energy.

Thank God, Archangel Michael, the healing angels and your guardian angel for their loving assistance and support.

Letting go of anger

Anger is a fiery, destructive emotion. If we suppress our anger it will turn into depression, a silent state, which is equally destructive.

As you have been working through the exercises in this book, you'll no doubt have felt your anger welling up on numerous occasions. Anger is energy and can be either released or transmuted into other forms of energy.

PRACTICAL WAYS TO TRANSMUTE ANGER

The seat of anger is the base chakra, which is red in colour, hence when we are angry "we see red". Anger energy springs from the originally neutral creative energy of the base. If you feel angry and you would like to transmute your anger energy into a more useful form, then utilise it to fuel some kind of physical process. This could be a wide range of activities, cleaning, doing the washing up, gardening or ironing your clothes, to mention just a few. As you get into action, you channel an otherwise destructive energy into something worthwhile. Sometimes anger can be a great spur to getting things done.

If you are not in the mood to work on transmuting anger, then here are some more physical ways, to release it.

When attempting some of these suggestions make sure that you are undisturbed and that you don't harm yourself or others in the process.

Ways to release anger

- Get hold of some pillows and punch them.
- Stomp around your house or garden
- Get into your car and scream.
- Go to a secluded spot in nature and scream.
- Do some strong physical exercise.
- Bang some drums (or pots and pans).

If you have been very angry, give yourself time to calm down and allow yourself to have a good cleansing cry; you'll feel much lighter afterwards.

All anger, be it at others or ourselves, needs to be released through forgiveness of the parties involved. All too often we hang on to our anger and internalise it for fear of speaking out and confronting the person who has caused it. Be aware that anger and blame are closely linked. You could keep the blame game going by constantly being angry with people, rooting yourself to the spot with this destructive behaviour.

Make the decision right now to first get hold of and then get rid of your anger.

If you have the clear intention to do so and the will to forgive yourself or anyone else involved, you'll succeed. To do so is love in action towards yourself.

Through the act of release and forgiveness, you allow more and more light into your life, making way to create the life you desire.

Now it is time to create a list of everyone you are angry with. Some of this anger may have been with you since childhood; some may be very recent – coming into being only a few minutes ago. No matter, list them all.

ANGER LIST EXERCISE

Think of all the people you are angry with and write down their names.

Next find out why you are angry with these people.

Here are some suggestions for your list.

I am angry at my father because _____

I am angry at my mother because _____

I am angry at my guardian because _____

I am angry at my friends because _____

I am angry at men because _____

I am angry at women because _____

I am angry at authority because _____

I am angry at God because _____

And now please take into contemplation what you are angry with yourself for.

I am angry with myself because _____

Please do some soul-searching and make the list longer

Now that we've established who the people are that you're angry with, you can use the following visualisation to voice your anger and then to forgive and heal it.

VOICING YOUR ANGER VISUALISATION

Make sure you allow at least 45 minutes for this exercise.

Take your phone of the hook and if possible turn off the doorbell.

Ask for divine assistance and give heartfelt thanks for what you'll receive.

Now take a deep breath in, aligning yourself with the divine will of God, releasing and letting go of all that is not love on the out-breath.

You feel that God and the angels are with you and all around you.

As you keep on breathing you become more and more relaxed.

Release and let go…

Relax and let go…

Allow your whole body to unwind…

In your own time, start to grow golden roots from the soles of your feet, down through the layers of mother earth into the middle of the earth, where they wrap themselves around a huge, beautiful rose quartz crystal.

With your next in-breath, you are drawing the soothing rose quartz crystal energy through your foot chakras into your body.

Allow this energy to rise up through the chakras filling them with rose-coloured light.

When you feel filled with light, imagine yourself sitting on a chair in a light, airy room.

The room is built of some kind of translucent material, which radiates a beautiful, soothing glow.

A group of healing angels is standing in attendance right behind you.

Now think of the person you are most angry with and ask the healing angels to fetch them into the room for you.

Soon they bring this person in and sit them down on the chair in front of you.

Now the healing angels are surrounding you both with a golden bubble of light.

The light is completely clear and will shield and protect you from any negative energy entering your auric field.

When you are ready tell the person opposite you why you are angry with them.

Once you have done that, get them to tell their side of the story.

Listen carefully to what they have to say, so as not to miss any of the important points they are trying to get across to you.

Remind yourself that this person did the best they could, according to their awareness, their abilities and circumstances they were in at the time.

Try to have compassion and understanding for their plight.

Once your conversation has finished, muster up as much love as you can and forgive the person concerned for what they did or did not do, as the case may be.

Then forgive yourself for the role you might have played and ask for your power to be returned to you from the other person.

The power energy is returned to you, neatly wrapped up in a parcel handed to you by the healing angels.

Take the energy and incorporate it back into your energy field, by placing the power parcel into your solar plexus.

If there is any power energy you have been retaining from this person, please give it back now.

Finally ask the healing angels to bless both of you, which they do instantly.

Say thank you to the person opposite you for coming to talk to you and ask the healing angels to escort them out of the room.

Thank the healing angels for their assistance and love.

Return to your present awareness and close down your chakras.

Visualise them as wooden gates made from solid oak, having sturdy locks with golden keys in them.

Starting from the crown chakra, firmly shut the gate, turning the key in the lock.

Repeat all the way through your chakras and finish at the base chakra.

When you are ready, imagine a cosy, sky-blue downy sleeping bag in front of you with a strong metallic zip. Now climb into it and zip it up.

You are completely safe and protected by the sky blue energy.

Give thanks to God and the healing angels for their loving support.

And give yourself a cuddle as well, you did great!

Congratulations for sticking with this exercise, as another influx of light has just flushed out more sticky energy from your auric field, leaving you lighter in body, mind, emotions and spirit!

You are now well on your way to loving yourself.

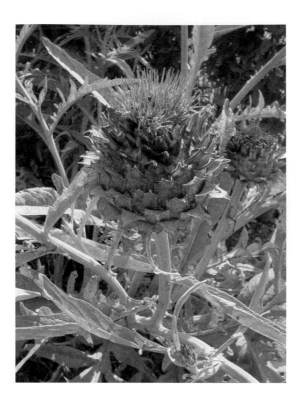

*"Holding anger is like grasping a hot coal with the intent of throwing it at
someone else; you are the one who gets burned."*
— *The Buddha*

Healing our inner child

As touched on in previous chapters, we all have an inner child within us, who is crying
out to be healed.

Our inner child is the part of us that has been abused or neglected at some time in our
childhood or teenage years. The emotional development of our inner child was hampered
and, in some cases, arrested at the time of the abuse.

Our emotional intelligence operates from the level of maturity of all the aspects of our
being. If our inner child is way behind in growing up emotionally, we'll behave from this
distorted energy within ourselves; in short our behaviour at times will be "childish".

We can easily observe the inner child in adults' behaviour and if we are sensitive
and look closely, we'll intuitively know at what age this inner child stopped maturing

emotionally and refused to grow up. (Try this out on your friends and family, you'll be surprised how accurate you are.)

Our inner child desires to be acknowledged and needs to be listened to so that it can grow up into an emotionally mature adult.

Our inner child has of course tried to give us messages all our adult lives, but we have for the most part ignored its pleas.

What our inner child is looking for is someone to mother and nurture it, to give it all it needs wholeheartedly.

Our need for approval, our emotional insecurities, and lack of self-confidence, self-worth and self-esteem often stem from this inner child aspect.

Now is the time for you to change all that by embracing and loving your inner child, giving it the chance to come along with you into mature adulthood.

The following visualisation will put you in touch with your inner child, its needs and desires. You'll be able to go a long way towards healing your inner child by using this energy process on an ongoing basis.

HEALING YOUR INNER CHILD VISUALISATION

Make sure that you are undisturbed for at least 45 minutes

Please get some hankies ready. You may need them.

Make yourself comfortable.

From your heart ask God, the healing angels and your guardian angel for their help with this important energy process. Give thanks for the wonderful outcome of your visualisation.

Now on the in-breath mentally ask to be aligned with God's divine will and your highest good and purpose.

On the out-breath release all that is not love.

As you do this, you become aware of the vibration of the healing angels around you.

The healing angels are giving you their loving energy to assist you with your visualisation.

Take a nice deep breath in…

Breathe out and release and let go of all your tensions and worries…

Repeat until you feel much calmer and more relaxed.

When you are ready, start to grow golden roots through the layers of the earth.

Soon you arrive at a large, sparkling rose quartz.

The rose quartz is glowing in a beautiful, nurturing and uplifting pink colour and you wrap your roots around it.

As you breathe in, you draw this special energy up via your roots into your foot chakras.

On the next in-breath you allow the nurturing vibration of the rose quartz to rise all the way up through all your chakras and flood them with pink light.

You now find yourself walking on a beautiful sandy beach.

There is no one around and you are enjoying your walk. Feel the sand beneath your feet; look at the sun high in the sky and delight at the turquoise colour of the sea.

As you are aware that you are on your way to meet your inner child, you get excited and start to walk a little faster.

You now leave the beach and a narrow path leads you up through the cliffs, past pretty pink coastal flowers on to a plateau on the top.

You arrive at this point and there is a lush green meadow spreading out ahead of you.

In the distance you can see a large, solitary oak tree.

You can just about make out that there is a little figure standing beneath it.

You know immediately that this little person is your inner child, standing there, waiting for you.

Automatically your feet start to run, carrying you closer and closer to meeting your inner child.

You can now see it waving its arms to you.

As you get nearer, you can also see that your inner child is crying.

Finally you arrive and straight away your inner child jumps into your arms, delighted to see you after all this time.

You give it the biggest, most loving hug of all, holding and caressing it.

Now the two of you sit down under the oak tree and you promise your inner child that from now on you will be its proper parent and will always be there for it, whenever it needs you.

Apologise to your inner child for the lack of attention you have given it over the years and explain why, as best you can, certain events happened to it.

Point out that the people involved in any kind of mental, emotional, sexual or physical abuse had been abused themselves at some time or other and where not capable of acting in a loving way. Apologise to the child that it had to go through these awful experiences.

As you talk to your inner child, while holding it tight, it is slowly starts to calm down.

Next ask your inner child what it would like you to do, to heal its little heart and make it happy again.

Your inner child might tell you that it wants some gifts, like a teddy bear or other toys that it never had and always wanted.

Or it might want to be taken out to play, to go to the movies, the park or the ice rink. Go and do some of those things together right away (This is an imaginary place and anything your child-self wants can appear instantly.)

Now your inner child is smiling happily and asking you to promise that you'll return for another visit soon.

You promise from your heart to return soon and give it another hug goodbye.

As you walk away, you can hear your inner child singing, while it is sitting happily under the oak tree.

Wander back through the green meadow allowing yourself to absorb the green healing energy of the grass.

Then climb down the cliff path until your arrive back at the beach.

As soon as you arrive there your run to the shore and as it is a nice day and nobody is around, you take off all your clothes and jump into the water.

Splash about or swim in the lovely warm ocean as long as you like.

Enjoy the experience.

When you are ready to come out, to your surprise you find that a set of fluffy white towels and a pile of brand new clothes have appeared on the shore, courtesy of the healing angels.

You are thrilled with these gifts. Dry yourself and get dressed.

Walk back along the beach until you arrive in your meditation room.

Once returned to present awareness, start to close down your chakras.

Imagine each one to be an open shell.

One by one, starting at the crown chakra close each shell until it is shut tight.

Carry on all the way down to your base chakra.

As you are finished, you become aware of a huge blue bubble of light in front of you.

Step into the bubble and feel yourself surrounded by its strong protective energy.

Thank God, the healing angels and your guardian angels for lending you a hand and assisting you with this energy process.

To make true progress with healing your inner child, you need to repeat this visualisation at least once a week to start with.

When you go back to your inner child in the meditation, bring a rucksack full of toys and other goodies you think your inner child might like. Sit down and play together.

Another part of the exercise is to do the practical things your child wants to experience in real life.

Go out and play and allow yourself to do the things your inner child is craving to do. You'll feel so much better for it.

Remember that denial is not getting you anywhere.

As you heal and nurture your inner child, you are allowing it to mature into the emotionally well-grounded, happy adult you, yourself, want to be.

Once the process has been completed, your inner child will merge with your adult self and you will become one; only then will you truly feel that you have "grown up".

You are now able to stand in your own power, independent of emotional needs and wants from times past.

You have learned to be your own inner parent utilising the unlimited love, power and strength from your higher God self to do so.

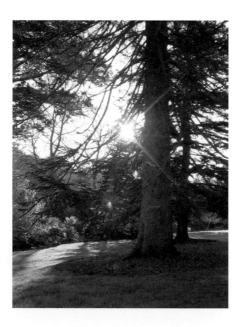

"One day your heart will take you to your Lover.
One day your soul will carry you to the Beloved.
Don't get lost in your pain, know that one day
your pain will become your cure."
—Rumi

How to gain self-confidence, self-worth and self-esteem

Most likely some of these issues will already have been either resolved or greatly improved by working with the exercises in this book.

I hope that the following insights will help you towards your goal of feeling happy and confident within yourself, no matter what the outside world is throwing at you.

The worst culprit, standing between us and acquiring self-confidence and self-esteem is our inner critic.

This is the conditioned voice within us, which is constantly telling us that we are no good at this, that or the other. It's sometimes called the critical inner parent, as the voice takes on the qualities of a parent who, in an unloving way, chips away at our confidence.

The critical inner parent is mostly based on a real life parent, guardian or teacher.

Someone close to us who has constantly criticised our every move can affect us profoundly, influencing the way we feel about ourselves for the rest of our life.

The comments our nearest and dearest have made will be etched into our subconscious mind and it is from there that they play havoc with our lives.

Moreover as we have been surrounded by criticism all our lives we'll have copied the behaviour of our parents and become critical of ourselves.

> *"The noble soul has reverence for itself"*
> *—Friedrich Nietzsche*

Often by just realising where the critical voices in your head come from, they can be released.

The following exercise will help you release and forgive those critical voices.

RELEASING THE CRITICAL INNER PARENT EXERCISE

Make sure that you have at least half an hour of quality time for yourself.

Ask for help from God and the healing angels and thank them for the positive outcome of your exercise.

Make yourself comfortable and ask your higher mind to help unlock what you would like to find out.

Now write a list of the critical comments your parents, guardians or other people close to you would have made.

Examples:

"This is just not good enough. Try harder."

"You are too stupid to do even the simplest task."

"You are too tall, too small, too fat, too thin, no one else in the family looks like this."

"You never do anything right."

Write your own list, leaving space after every criticism.

When you have done this, write a positive affirmation opposite the negative criticism.

Example:

"What I have done is just fine and good enough for me."

"I am bright and intelligent and able to do anything I want."

"I am perfect the way I am, never mind what anyone else in the family looks like."

"I do the best I can and that is ok with me."

Now forgive and let go of the people who have criticised you.

You are able to do this, as you are aware that any critical parent was in turn criticised by their parents or people close to them.

Next think about what you are criticising yourself for and write it down.

Example:

"I should have been able to do this much better…"

"I am never going to get things right in my life…"

"I have got a slow mind…"

"I have got an ugly body…"

"I never have anything interesting to say…"

Please carry on with this list.

When the list is complete, write a positive affirmation opposite the negative self-criticism, as in the last exercise.

Go through the items on your list one by one and from the bottom of your heart allow the light of forgiveness to wash away all the negative self-criticism you have stored up.

Release and clear it once and for all.

Finally ask God and the healing angels to bless all involved including yourself.

Give thanks for the love and support you have received.

As you release your critical inner parent, the cause of your lack of self-confidence, self-esteem and sense of self-worth will become apparent.

Remember that we are in control of our lives, that we are the one who chooses how to feel and how not to feel today. We can decide to feel joy and leave the old emotional baggage behind.

We are also the one who chooses how to react to certain people and situations. Will we choose to react with love and have a happy day or will we allow ourselves to fall back into old conditioned behaviour patterns, reacting from fear and hate – and have a miserable one? It's our choice!

The positive energy of our divinity has only been suppressed by our conditioned thinking and behaviour: at the core of our being we are perfect, this means that each of us is naturally self-confident, full of self-esteem and self-worth.

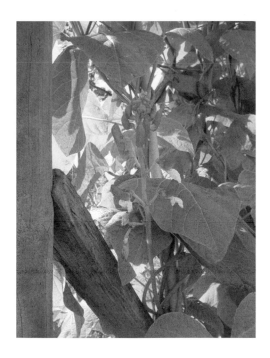

"Be a lamp to yourself. Be your own confidence.
Hold to the truth within yourself, as to the only truth."
—The Buddha

Part 6:
Body matters

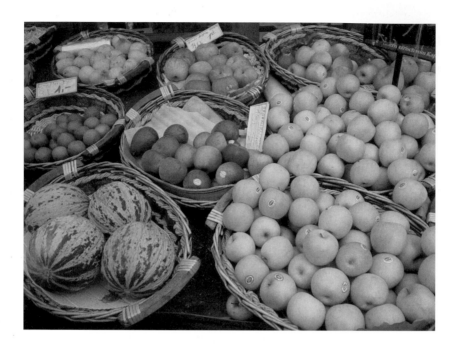

"We are shaped and fashioned by what we love."
— *Johann Wolfgang Goethe*

The body, the temple of the soul

We've travelled together from the God plane, through the realms of spirit – mind and emotions – and now are arriving at the realm of the physical body, the densest of the energy bodies. There the light of God within vibrates at its lowest level, the physical body being the manifestation of the finer energies, namely of the thoughts and feelings we have about ourselves, manifested into matter.

I hope that on our journey through the layers of awareness many "mental and emotional buttons" have been pressed and that the negative energies of outmoded thought forms and belief systems have been released by the truckload!

We have learned: It's not necessarily the food that is fattening but the thoughts, the negative beliefs and the expectations we have about the food.

- It's not others who make us unhappy, but our own reaction to their behaviour.

- We have choices and we are free to choose again and again and again…

- Forgiveness is the greatest transformational tool of all.

- Unconditional love is the ultimate power and the ultimate reality rolled together into one.

- We truly are all-powerful beings of light, dwelling in a physical body.

- We are co-creators with God and we are creating our own reality. With every thought we think, every word we speak, every outburst of emotion and every action we take, we define who and what we are. We now have the golden opportunity to show our true colours. Let's take this blessed chance to be a true sparkling diamond in the heart of God.

- The choice is ours as stated by the law of free will.

- We can carry on abusing the divine God-given gifts that have been so liberally bestowed on to us or we can love, cherish and make good use of these gifts from now on.

As the body truly is the temple of the soul, it pays to look after it. The more time we are able to spend in this splendid abode, the more chance we have of attaining enlightenment in our present lifetime.

The healthier our body is and the happier we are within it, the longer we'll live. Our aim therefore must be to ensure that our body stays in the best possible shape, while our soul is still ensconced within it.

There are various ways to assist the body to gain and maintain maximum health; most of these options are very simple to follow, but often take quite a lot of willpower to implement successfully.

PRACTICAL TIPS FOR LONGEVITY:

- Have plenty of rest and take power naps.

- Get a good night's sleep.

- Take regular exercise, such as Yoga, Tai chi and Chi Gung which also allows maximum light to come into the body by utilising the divine breath.

- Spend as much time as possible in nature.

- Be aware of breathing, and practise relaxation techniques when under stress.

- Meditate regularly; this might take the form of contemplation such as painting, dancing or walking in nature.

- Love and respect the body and don't stretch it to its limits.

- Drink plenty of mineral water.

- Eat fresh foods, mainly nuts, fruits and vegetables.

- Bless all food and drinks you consume.

- Look for the best in everything and everyone.

- Enjoy the small things in life.

- Live every day as if it's your last.

The illusion of death

The worst fear for most of us is the fear of death. The higher reality is quite different. In the journey of the soul from source to matter and back again, losing a material body is not something to fear, as our Soul, our essence, our consciousness does not and cannot die.

As we release this fear of death and dwell more and more in God's love and trust, some surprising things happen.

There are some people amongst us who are:

a) the "super young" who look 10 to 20, or even 30, years younger than their biological age

b) the "super old" who live to a very old age of about 120 or so and stay in very good mental and physical shape

c) the ancient ones, who walk amongst us but are hundreds of years old; this is a fact to which I can personally testify having met a Tibetan master in the Himalayas, whom I firmly believe, was indeed ancient

How is this possible?

The reason is simply that energy follows thought. All of these people have a youthful outlook on life and are young at heart into the bargain; their thinking, attitudes and behaviour are that of a mature, yet youthful person who takes an interest in the joys of life, keeping flexible and agile in this way. These people live "for the now and in the now" utilising their power of positive thought, which automatically maintains their bodies in good health.

The higher reality is that God is pure love, love which is without condition; God never has and never will judge us, therefore there is nothing to fear in returning to God via death.

God has given us the gift of free will, allowing us to make our own way back to heaven and, by the same gift, to create our own version of paradise on earth.

God created this universe for our benefit, to give us the opportunity to become conscious of who we truly are, namely a spark of His divinity, all powerful, perfect and whole in every way.

We may have descended so far into matter that we've forgotten our origins, but we are now awakening from our slumber of many lifetimes.

A new and glorious reality is dawning, one where we have within ourselves power freely available to us and have the God-given right to use it for the benefit of ourselves and all creatures on mother earth. If we focus on love, we draw life-force to us. If we focus on fear, life-force is drawn from us. Therefore to prolong healthy, active life, we need simply turn our thoughts to love.

Energy follows thought and our thoughts create our reality.

If we choose lively, joyful, vibrant loving thoughts, our bodies will follow suit.

Allow your thoughts to be divinely inspired; allow the full blast of divine light to transmute all negativity throughout every fibre of your being!

To be able to clearly manifest a positive reality, a reality of freedom from the fear of death, we need to clear our subconscious of all fear.

Fear of death and its links to eating

Somewhere deep inside, most of us seem to believe that something terrible could happen to us at any time, that a powerful force outside of us has the power to snatch us away from life at any given moment – something we have no control over whatsoever. This force is portrayed as God. Death is the ultimate fear; we fear death as the outcome of many, even minor, life events. As the body always obeys our thoughts, it takes our fears of death very seriously and wants to protect us by sending hunger signals to the brain. We eat to feel safe and protected, fat is the ultimate protection from any harm that might come to us, even if we're not aware of it. The body does it all for us automatically.

To be our perfect body-shape we need to lose our fear of death.

As we learn to listen to our soul, speaking to us via our intuition and our emotions we learn to trust God more and more.

As we now have begun to search for the light, the light will reveal itself to us little by little. We will be able to perceive the divine love and light of God operating in everything and through everything. And an inner knowing will grow that God truly is walking by our side every minute of the day and night.

We are now free to let go of the false beliefs in a death caused by outside forces and move into our own power. As soon as we do so, the body is able to release the protection it has created for us, which is no longer needed, since we now feel safe from within our own divine God-self.

The reality of immortality

Now let us move on to some powerful affirmations. The most potent statement we can make is that we are immortal beings of light incarnated in a physical body, thereby acknowledging our divinity. The more we affirm this truth, the more we become established in it and the more natural and right it will feel to us.

With every affirmation we are drawing God's love into our being, grounding and anchoring the divine light in our soul.

And so the divine spark within grows and expands…

IMMORTALITY AFFIRMATIONS

Please make this exercise into a special occasion.

Make sure you have at least 30 minutes to yourself.

Light a candle or some incense and make yourself comfortable.

Now ask God, the healing angels, your guardian angels and all other beings of light to be with you and assist you with these affirmations.

Give thanks from your heart for the love you are about to receive.

Now read the following affirmations out loud 9 times:

I, _____ , *am an immortal being of light*

And so be it.

And so be it.

And so be it.

I AM THE I AM.

I AM THE I AM.

I AM THE I AM.

I, _____ , *completely trust in the power of an all-loving God.*

I, _____ , *am wholly protected by the divine power of God.*

I, _____ , *totally trust in a supportive universe.*

I, _____ , *have the power over my own destiny.*

I, _____ , *now feel safe to let go of any surplus weight.*

I, _____ , *now trust God with my highest good.*

I, _____ , *hand my body over to God's care and safekeeping.*

And so be it.

And so be it.

And so be it.

I AM THE I AM.

I AM THE I AM.

I AM THE I AM.

This was a huge completion for you and I can hear the angels sing with joy at your success!

Give yourself a cuddle for your brilliant efforts.

Give a million thanks to God and the realms of light for their unwavering support on your journey into the light of your divine self.

> **"The snow goose need not bathe to make itself white.**
> **Neither need you do anything but be yourself."**
> **—Lao Tse**

Making room for more light

To keep the body the temple of the soul in pristine condition, it needs to be cleansed and cleared of all negativity on a regular basis.

On the physical levels of course, we do this through having regular showers, and, as the element of water represents the emotions, as we shower we are also releasing emotional tensions from the body. Water also helps to clear and purify the magnetic field, the part of the aura closest to the physical body, which becomes clogged up with negative thought-forms along with electromagnetic pollution from computers, television, microwave ovens, electricity pylons, telecommunication masts, mobile phones, etc. A contaminated magnetic field leads to toxicity, which in turn brings on tiredness and headaches, and may induce states of anger and fear and feeling unwell. If we start to feel tired, besides practising the following very effective guided imagery, it helps to rub the body with a sea salt preparation and then take a shower. The salt will absorb negativity and the water will wash it away, supporting the emotional body in the process. We'll feel fresh and rejuvenated after this cleansing treatment.

As the crown chakra receives the incoming divine energy, washing the hair regularly is beneficial; this also clears the head if we have a headache or feel stressed by mental activity.

Now let me introduce you to a thorough, highly effective visualisation that will clear any toxins out of your chakras, your auric field and your entire physical body.

This exercise uses the colour black, which might at first be alarming to you, as black has negative esoteric associations. No worries though, as black is the perfect vibration to absorb negativity. We first take the black energy into our chakras, our auric field and our physical body, then flush it out with brilliant white light.

The black vibration, having absorbed all the negativity present in the body, flows out of the energy system into mother earth where Gaia kindly transmutes all the negative waste into earthlight.

There are many benefits to be gained from this exercise.

It will help you to:

- Clear your chakras

- Clear your auric field

- Release muscle tension

- Cleanse your organs

- Cleanse your blood

- Get rid of diseased cells

- Boost your immune system

The exercise might also be beneficial for a variety of ailments. However, it's not intended as a substitute for medical treatment, although it may be used in conjunction with treatments prescribed by your doctor.

THE ULTIMATE BODY CLEANSE VISUALISATION

For this very thorough exercise please allow an hour to begin with. Later on, with practice, you'll be able to do this visualisation much faster, in approximately 20 minutes.

Ask God, the healing angels and beings of light for their aid with this cleansing process and thank them for the brilliant results you are about to achieve.

Make sure that you won't be disturbed

Make yourself comfortable.

As you take a deep breath in, mentally align yourself with the divine will of God and the highest good for yourself.

On the out-breath release and let go of all that does not serve you anymore.

You can feel God's love and light enveloping you and you feel safe and sound.

Now with every breath you take you feel more and more relaxed…

All the tensions you are holding in your body are draining away from you…

Release and let go…

In your own good time, start to grow golden roots from the soles of your feet down through the layers of the earth; where at the earth's core they arrive at a pool of beautiful black energy.

You may visualise the black energy as either a very dark or a greyish shade of black. Your higher self will intuitively show you the right tone, or you might get a strong sense of the colour if you are not able to visualise but please remember the darker the black vibration the more negative energy it will be able to absorb.

Make the black energy as dense as you like. It could vary from a fairly thick syrup-like substance to a much thinner fluid.

As you dip your hollow golden roots into the black fluid you find that it feels nice and soothing and is just the right temperature for you.

When you are ready, take a deep breath in and draw the black vibration all the way into your foot chakras, from there allow it to permeate every single muscle fibre in your body.

As you exhale, breathe out all that you are ready to release and which no longer serves you.

Start with your feet and work all the way up to your jaw and facial muscles.

With every breath you take, another group of muscles absorbs the black vibration.

Do this slowly, moving from your feet, to your calve muscles, to your thigh muscles, the muscles on your buttocks, your abdominal muscles, your pectoral muscles, your back and shoulder muscles, your biceps and lower arm muscles, the muscles in your hands and fingers and finally your neck, your jaw and facial muscles.

If you have muscle pain or suffer from muscle spasms in specific areas focus more black energy into those areas.

Now that all your muscles have absorbed the black vibration, refocus your awareness on your golden roots in the black pool.

Take a deep breath in and allow the black vibration to rise up into your foot chakras and now allow it to fill every single nerve and nerve ending in your body.

Again work your way through your whole body all the way up to the top of your head, imagining the billions of little tiny nerves and nerve endings absorbing this beneficial black vibration.

If you are aware that you are holding nervous tension in specific parts of your body, please direct more black energy to these parts.

Remember to always release and let go on the out-breath.

Next focus on your roots again, take a big breath in, allow the black vibration to flow upwards into your foot chakras and now allow it to permeate every single bone in your body, starting with the tiny bones in your toes.

As you keep on breathing, draw the black energy into your foot bones, your fibula, your thigh bones and up into your hipbones, your pelvic girdle, and from there into your spine.

With another in-breath, you see the black vibration flow into the bones of your rib cage and then into your pectoral girdle, your shoulder bones, down into the bones of your arms, hands and fingers.

At the next in-breath allow the black energy to continue up your spine into the bones of your neck and finally into your skull.

Pay particular attention to past injuries, broken bones or places in your body where you experience bone ache, directing an extra dose of black energy to these areas.

When you are ready, become aware of your roots again, take a deep breath in and draw the black vibration all the way up via your foot chakras into the organs in your body, starting with your genital organs, filling them with black vibration, then moving on to your bladder, your colon and intestines, your kidneys, your pancreas and spleen, your stomach, your liver and gall bladder, your heart, your lungs, from there to your bronchial tubes, then up into your sensory organs, mouth, eyes, ears and nose and last but not least, fill your brain with plenty of black vibration.

If you experience pain in any specific organ or have a disease related to one of them, administer an extra dose of black energy to that part of your body.

In your own good time refocus again on your golden roots dangling in the pool of black vibration and when you are ready take a deep breath in and bring that energy all the way up into your foot chakras and from there distribute the black vibration to all of your blood cells.

First visualise all your white blood cells absorbing the black vibration.

Next visualise all your red blood cells absorbing the black vibration.

Now ask for any diseased or abnormal cells to show up and fill those with a high dose of black energy.

Remind yourself to release and let go on every out-breath.

When you have done that, return your attention again to your roots, take a deep breath and bring the black energy back up into your foot chakras and from there all the way up your legs into your base chakra.

Fill your base chakra and your gonads, which are associated with it, with the black vibration.

When you have done that, move on to your sacral chakra and your adrenal glands and fill them with the black energy.

From there move to your solar plexus and your pancreas and allow the black energy to penetrate them.

Next allow the black energy to travel up into your heart chakra and your thymus gland, permeating it with the black vibration.

Remember to always release and let go on the out-breath.

As you have now traversed from the lower chakras into the higher ones, the black energy coming up will not be as intense anymore.

Now, in your own good time, move on to your throat chakra and the thyroid gland.

Next on the list are your third eye chakra and the pituitary gland. Finally bring the black energy up into your crown chakra and the pineal gland.

And for one last time refocus again on your roots in the pool of black energy, take a deep breath and as you draw it up through the soles of your feet, allow it to fill the seven layers of your auric field, starting at the layer next to your body.

Simply see the black vibration filling layer after layer, becoming lighter and less dense as you imagine moving towards the outside of your auric field.

When you have done that, imagine that you have plug holes placed on the soles of your feet, your foot chakras, the palms of your hands, your palm chakras, and at every single chakra: the crown chakra, the third eye chakra, the throat chakra, the heart chakra, the solar plexus chakra, the sacral chakra and the base chakra.

Withdraw your golden roots from the pool of black vibration and bring them up through the layers of the earth.

After you have moved up a few layers, you come across an ancient fossilised oak tree trunk and you firmly wrap your golden roots around it.

Now you become aware of the presence of a strong white light.

As you look up with your inner eye, you see a ball of white light above your head and a huge beam of light emerging from it.

When you are ready, take a deep breath in, while mentally opening all the plug holes in your chakras and allow the powerful beam of light to enter the top of your head. Starting with your jaw and facial muscles allow it to flush away all the negative energy trapped by the black vibration from the muscles of your body.

On the out-breath, the murky energy is expelled through all the open plugholes in your major and minor chakras.

You can make the diameter of the plugholes as large as you like, so that the negative energy is able to exit swiftly.

The waste quickly flows into the ground and is transmuted courtesy of Gaia into earthlight.

As you breathe in, you see another beam of white light flowing into the next set of muscles, and on the out-breath you witness the negative energy rushing out of the plugholes into the ground.

Move all the way down your body releasing and letting go of the negative energies held in your muscle groups, administering an extra dose of light to aching or injured muscles or muscle groups.

On the next in-breath, allow the beam of brilliant white light to flow via your crown chakra into all of the nerves and nerve endings in your body.

See the white light carrying away all negativity, which is released through the plugholes situated in your energy centres, flowing away into the earth, on the out-breath.

Start with the tiny nerve endings on your scalp, then your facial nerves and move all the way down your body, not forgetting to especially cleanse any areas where you know you hold nervous tension.

When you are ready, take another deep breath in, directing the brilliant beam of white light into the bones of your body, starting with your skull bone and in your own time move all the way down through all the bones of your skeleton.

As you breathe out, the waste energy rushes out of the plugholes situated in your chakras and is absorbed by mother earth.

Bring an extra beam of white light into any breaks or injuries you might have had.

With the next breath in, you bring the shaft of powerful white light into your brain, the first organ of your body, releasing, on the out-breath, all negative vibrations which swiftly flows out of the plugholes of your chakras.

Carry on this way through all your organs all the way down to your genitals, releasing and letting go and watching the negativity being absorbed into the ground.

Allow an extra beam of strong white light to flow into any diseased or painful organs and watch as the negative vibrations are carried out of your body and seep into the ground to be transmuted.

In your own time, take in another deep breath and drawing the brilliant beam of white light to flow into the top of your head, allowing it to flow into all of your red blood cells. Push out any negative energy, which then exits through the plugholes located in your chakras as you breathe out.

Next on the list are your white blood cells.

Breathe in the brilliant white light and watch as the negative energy leaves your white *blood cells.*

With another big breath bring another shaft of white light into your body and direct it to any invading, diseased or abnormal cells.

Observe, on the out-breath, how the white light carries them straight out of your body and mother earth transmutes the now dead cells into earth light.

Repeat several times as this part of the exercise will greatly boost your immune system.

Now, as you take yet another deep breath, allow the brilliant white light to flow into your crown chakra and let the light flood the pineal gland as you breathe out.

Move on to your third eye chakra and the pituitary gland again filling both with powerful white light on the in-breath and expelling all negative energy via your plugholes on the out-breath.

Next comes your throat chakra and thyroid gland, as you allow the white light to enter your energy system on the in-breath, releasing all negativity out of your throat chakra and thyroid gland, on the out-breath.

As you breathe in now, bring an extra powerful beam of white light into your heart chakra and the thymus gland, watching as all negative energy is expelled via the plugholes on the out-breath.

You'll need to focus on the light more intensely as you move down the chakras into the lower vibrational levels, as the energy there is denser and more difficult to shift.

Now it's time for your solar plexus centre and your pancreas to be cleared.

Breathe in the white light and see all negative energy expelled on the out-breath.

When you are ready, take the next big breath in and direct a strong beam of white light into your sacral chakra and your adrenal glands.

Observe as the white light clears away all negative energy from the area, which escapes through the plugholes and soon disappears in the ground.

Now, with a big effort, breathe in deeply and bring an enormous beam of light all the way from your crown chakra into your base chakra and your gonads.

As you breathe out, you see the murky energy shooting out of your plugholes and draining away into the earth.

Now that your chakras and corresponding glands are all filled with brilliant light and clear of all psychic debris, we can move on to your auric field.

When you are ready, imagine the beam of light turning into a huge silver-coloured, metallic showerhead and as you breathe in, you give the signal for the heavenly power shower to be turned on.

Immediately masses of brilliant white light flood the layers of your auric field, taking away all psychic debris that was stored within it, as you breathe out.

With every breath you take, the brilliant white light will clear another layer of your aura.

Start with the layer next to your body and work your way outwards until your aura is filled with light and all negative energy has been washed away and released into the ground.

You are now ready to unwrap your golden roots from the fossilised oak tree trunk and bring them up through the layers of the earth, leaving them in a few inches deep for extra grounding; this is especially important after the powerful exercise you have just been through.

Give a big heartfelt thank you for all the love, light and help you have received with this visualisation.

You might want to rest for a while after this energy process and then drink some mineral water and maybe have a bite to eat to ground yourself even further.

You have just achieved a wonderful cleansing and will feel much better for it on many levels.

(This meditation is a variation of the theme taught to me by my former spiritual mentor David Cousins. Thank you David for all you have given to me.)

Body love

Finally we have arrived at the densest level of our being, at the level of the physical body, the place where conditioned thinking and beliefs have manifested into flesh.

First the mind must be healed, then the emotions, as the body is the product of both our mind patterns and how we feel about ourselves.

As the body is the final and lowest vibrational level of light manifestation, it is also the last level in which true release and healing will take place.

Our next task is to help our bodies to receive our new positive thoughts and feelings, by releasing old patterns from our body-consciousness.

The body truly is a miracle, don't you think?

To have the ability to think wonderfully creative thoughts, to utter words of comfort, to feel the emotions of true love, to perform random acts of kindness, to be able to behold the wonders of the world around you, to hear the birds singing in the sky, to be able to smell the roses and to taste delicious foods is truly a divine gift.

The body is a divine instrument given to us by God to enjoy life and fulfil our destiny on planet earth.

Whatever that destiny might be, it needs to be reached with the body, the temple of the soul, intact.

How much thought do we give to the body?

Not much, I am certain. The body is seen as a commodity, like a car, although I have to point out that most cars are looked after very well, loved and cherished and even washed and polished on Sundays, which is much more attention than we lavish onto our bodies under normal circumstances.

As we carry on abusing our bodies they desperately try to communicate the effects of this mistreatment to us. There are many signs, such as constant tiredness, flu-like symptoms, recurring head or backaches, to name just a few of the most common ones.

Do we listen to our bodies? No, we do not; we just carry on in exactly the same way.

We would not do this to our car; we'd take it to be repaired. Most people see even the tiniest scratch in the paintwork as a disaster.

However the body eventually, not having been taken into consideration and listened to, starts to fight back, by producing "dis-ease". This means that by now the body really could be very ill at ease.

The greatest healer of all is the power of love. Once we learned to apply the medicine of love and light to the body, not only will we heal many psychosomatic illnesses, but we will also release extra weight far more easily and quickly, and, in the case of under eating we will put on the weight we so much desire. Once we have shown it our unconditional love and appreciation the body, will happily co-operate with us and a state of balance will be achieved much more easily. The power of unconditional love from our own hearts will wash away all ills.

Your body is craving your personal attention and in the next exercise you will give it just that, the love, care, attention and gratitude it so much deserves.

You are a co-creator with God and have the power to transform your body into the perfect one you have always dreamt of.

GRATITUDE AND BODY-HEALING VISUALISATION

As this is an in-depth exercise, please allow an hour to be able to do it successfully. Your body is worthy of your attention!

Please have pen and paper to hand.

As we are going to be thanking each of the areas of your body associated with the chakras, here is a list of their main associations:

> BASE CHAKRA: Feet, legs, hips, skeleton, large intestine and organs of elimination including kidneys and bladder, organs of reproduction, muscular system

SACRAL CHAKRA: Adrenal glands, pelvic girdle

SOLAR PLEXUS CHAKRA: Liver, gall bladder, spleen, pancreas, stomach, small intestine

HEART CHAKRA: Heart, lungs, breasts, circulatory system and blood, skin, thymus gland

THROAT CHAKRA: voice box, tonsils, nose and mouth, airways, thyroid gland

THIRD EYE CHAKRA: Eyes, ears, pineal gland, lymphatic system

CROWN CHAKRA: Brain, nervous system, pituitary gland

Call on God, the healing angels, your guardian angel and the beings of light to support you in this task. Give thanks for what you are about to receive.

Ensure that you will not be disturbed and make yourself comfortable.

As you take a deep breath in, you can sense that you are enveloped in a force field of love and light.

You feel safe and cared for by the heavens.

As you breathe out ,release and let go of all that does not serve you anymore.

On the next in-breath, align yourself mentally with the divine will of God, your highest purpose and highest good.

Release all that is not love on the out-breath.

As you carry on breathing, you start to feel more and more relaxed.

Slowly your muscles release all tension…

Your mind starts to quieten down…

Your breathing slows down and you feel much calmer.

In your own good time you start to grow golden roots from the soles of your feet down through the layers of the earth until you arrive at a large granite boulder.

You now firmly wrap your golden roots around it, feeling perfectly anchored in the process.

Next you become aware of a golden light surrounding you.

This is the golden universal healing light, which is enveloping you in its protective, nurturing and healing vibration.

You take a deep breath in and allow the light, entering through your crown chakra, to flood your whole chakra system and your auric field all at once with its pure golden vibration.

As it does so, a sense of well-being spreads through your whole body.

Breathe in the golden light, then release and let go on the out-breath.

Now, physically, put your hands over your base chakra with fingertips touching each other.

Sit still for a little while and just be.

Now, from your heart, mustering all the love you've got to give, thank the parts of your body connected to this area for all the hard work they have done for you in this lifetime.

Thank your legs for carrying you, your feet for walking, etc.

Thank your arms and hands for doing the work you need to do.

Go on to thank any part of your body associated with your base chakra…

Give extra special thanks to any diseased areas in the region of your base chakra.

You will sense how grateful your body is for your acknowledgement.

Next apologise for any abuse you might have caused this area of your body whether knowingly or unknowingly, and ask your body to forgive you.

Now give yourself a cuddle and forgive yourself for what you did or think you should've done.

Take another deep breath of golden healing light and allow the light to flow into your crown chakra, from there into your third eye chakra, on to your throat chakra and into your heart chakra. From there let the golden healing vibration flow on into your lungs, filling your lungs with light then on into your bronchis and down your upper arms, elbows, lower arms into the palms of your hands, where two minor chakras are situated.

Mentally open the palm chakras as you would open a floodgate and allow the golden healing light to flow through your palms, which are resting over your base chakra, and straight into your body.

Your body is very happy indeed to receive this lovely healing.

Spend about five minutes doing this, carrying on breathing in the golden light and releasing and letting go on the out-breath.

You will find that you know intuitively when this area of your body has absorbed enough light.

(Some parts of your body may need more light than others.)

To complete the work with this chakra, ask the area of your body you are working with if there is anything else you can do for it.

Your body might answer you by showing you images of what it desires from you or it might communicate to you through flashes of inspirations. You might even hear it talking to you.

Your body might ask you to carry out specific physical activities, like sports and exercise, or to eat certain foods, drink more water, take more rest and so on.

Promise your body that you will do the best you can to fulfil its wishes.

When you have completed this energy process with your base chakra, please move on to the next one up, the sacral chakra and in your own good time repeat the exact same process of:

- *Giving thanks to your body for the life-long services rendered to you unconditionally*

- *Apologising for the abuse you have inflicted on it*

- *Asking for forgiveness from your body*

- *Forgiving yourself for what you have done or failed to do for your body*

- *Administering self-healing*

- *Finding out what else your body needs*

Repeat this energy process all the way up through your chakras to your crown chakra.

Remember to apply some extra healing to painful or diseased areas of your body and to continue breathing in the golden light, allowing all that is not love to be released on the out-breath.

As this is a long exercise, you might have forgotten what your body has told you at the base chakra level by the time you have reached the crown chakra, so please make a written note of what each area of the body has to say to you at each stage.

When you have gone through your whole body in this manner, start to slowly unwrap your golden roots from the granite boulder and continue bringing them up through the layers of mother earth, leaving them in just a few inches, for extra grounding.

Now you are ready to close down your chakras, starting at the crown chakra.

Imagine them to be wooden gates, made from solid oak, having sturdy locks with golden keys in them.

Close the gates one by one behind you, turning the golden keys firmly in their locks, finishing with the base chakra.

In your own good time, ask your guardian angel to hand you the cloak of protection, which your angel puts around you immediately.

The cloak, made from heavy sky blue velvet, is lined with gorgeous golden satin and is full length with a big hood and long sleeves.

It fits your perfectly, made in heaven just for you, and you now feel safe and protected.

Give a big thank you to God, the healing angels, the beings of light and your guardian angel for their love and assistance with this healing meditation.

Reminder: Do not forget to carry out your body's requests.

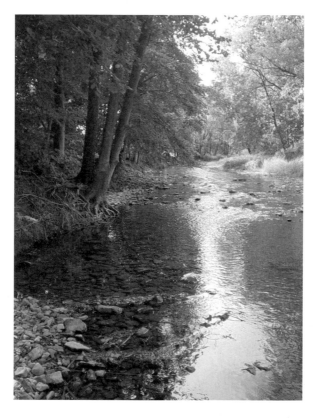

"Patience is the companion of wisdom."
—St.Augustine

Releasing ourselves from all that is not love

To bring ourselves truly into the here and now is a difficult task at the best of times, as old patterns, habits and outmoded belief systems try to drag us forever back into the past.

To be fully present in the now and have all the creative power we need to achieve our goals at our fingertips is the ultimate aim.

The following visualisation will greatly aid you with your goal to be in control of your destiny right here and right now.

Working with the violet flame is one of the most magical and potent transformational tools that has been gifted to us by divine dispensation.

The violet flame has the ability to transmute negative energy into positive energy, and to raise consciousness into a higher frequency. It helps to accelerate spiritual development and to release negative karma and burn off old karmic ties.

THE VIOLET FLAME VISUALISATION

Please allow about 20 minutes for this visualisation.

Make sure that you will not be disturbed and make yourself comfortable.

Ask God, the healing angels and especially Archangel Michael to look after you, to guide and protect you during this exercise.

Give thanks for the magical results you will achieve.

You might experience physical heat while you are doing this exercise, which is quite natural with this powerful meditation.

Take a deep breath in, and mentally align yourself with the divine will of God for your highest good and highest purpose and that of all sentient beings on planet earth.

On the out-breath release all that is not love.

While you carry on breathing, you become aware that God, the healing angels and Archangel Michael are enveloping you in their love and light.

As you take another deep breath in, your body starts to relax, and all tension drains away as you breathe out.

When you are ready, grow golden roots from the soles of your feet, down through the layers of mother earth until you arrive at a large chunk of amethyst crystal.

You wrap your roots around this beautiful amethyst and are safely grounded.

You are now aware that the energy around you has turned into a luminous white light with a pearly sheen to it.

As you look with your third eye, you can make out the colours of the rainbow in a pastel hue shining through the luminous pearly white light.

And as you breathe in, the energy washes through you in a big, but gentle wave of vibration, starting from your crown chakra and flowing right through into your base chakra.

Take another breath in and see the luminous white energy forming a bubble of light around you.

This is a bubble of special protection.

Now ask from the point of your I AM consciousness, that is, from your higher divine self, for the dispensation of the violet flame to be given to you.

As soon as you have done that, you become aware of a violet flame growing beneath your foot chakras.

With every breath you take, the intensity and size of the violet flame increases, forming a column of violet fire around you.

As you breathe out, release and let go of all that is not love.

The violet flame is assisting you greatly with this process and the more you focus on the flame, which represents the power of love and light, the stronger it will become.

Keep focussing on your breathing and mentally ask for the violet flame to dissolve the cause, effect, record and memory of your own and others negative karmic deeds, through all times and all dimensions of reality.

Believe that this will be done, by the grace of the Almighty.

Allow the violet fire to now enter your auric field and move into your chakras, clearing and cleansing them of all residue of negative energy.

Keep on breathing in love and light and releasing all that is no longer serving you on the out-breath.

As the violet fire rises up through your energy centres and at the same time through the layers of the auric field, it burns away and transmutes everything that is not light and does not serve your highest purpose anymore.

(If you find the violet fire too strong ask Archangel Michael, who is standing by you, to turn down the intensity.)

Stay in the force field of the violet fire as long as it feels comfortable and necessary to do so.

When you feel that you are done for now, ask Archangel Michael to assist you in extinguishing the fire.

You watch as the flames recede, become smaller and smaller and eventual disappearing into the earth beneath your feet.

Now unwrap your golden roots from the amethyst rock and slowly bring them up through the layers of the earth, leaving them a few inches deep in the ground, to give you extra anchoring for the rest of the day.

Please note: It is very important to keeps your roots earthed following this process. This is a very high-energy exercise, which might leave you ungrounded if you don't leave your roots in.

When you are ready, close down your chakras, starting with the crown chakra. Imagine them to be heavy silver trap doors, held open by strong silver chains.

As you let go of the silver chains the trap door shuts with a mighty clang.

Repeat all the way down to your base chakra, firmly shutting all of the trap doors behind you.

That done you are ready to protect yourself.

See a giant open seashell in front of you, its mother of pearl interior glowing with a beautiful translucent sheen.

When you are ready, step into the shell, which gently closes around you, protecting you with its luminous, yet strong vibrational energy.

Thank God, Archangel Michael, the healing angels and all the beings of light for the love and assistance they've given you.

Drink a glass of mineral water and possibly eat something grounding after this energy process.

Have some quiet time before you resume your everyday activities.

"Paradise is where I am"
— Voltaire

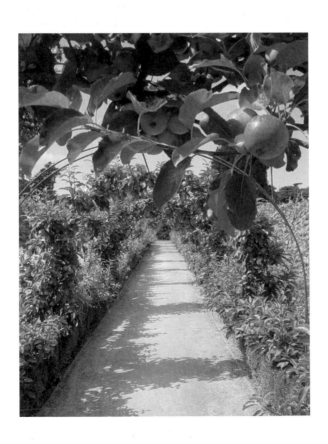

Part 7:
Food for the soul, mind, emotions and body

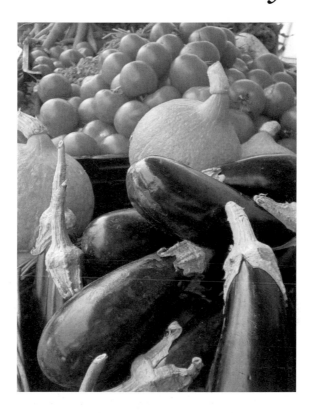

*"Keeping your body healthy is an expression of gratitude to the whole cosmos
– the trees, the clouds, everything"*
—*Thich Nhat Hanh*

Food for the soul

*"If you keep your heart immersed always in the ocean of divine love, your heart
is sure to remain full to overflowing with the waters of divine love."*
—*Ramakrishna*

Our soul, ensconced within the chamber of our heart has suffered much through the
many lifetimes it has been journeying into matter on our behalf.

It has been, and still to this moment is, working tirelessly to help guide us into the light of our own true divine nature, constantly communicating to us through the language of the emotions.

Most of all it is trying to impress on us that God loves us so much, far beyond our comprehension. Our soul endeavours to communicate to us that we are safe in the universe God has created for us and that no matter what we will always return to our divine homeland, into the bosom of our father/mother God.

Even in physical death our unique divine essence, our soul, can never be lost and will live on in all eternity.

To enable our soul to "keep up the good work", it needs to be fed, just as our body needs to be nourished. Our daily lives do not provide much soul food, so we must make an extra effort on our soul's behalf.

Here are some suggestions as to how to "feed" your soul. The Following was originally a Zen exercise.

PRACTISING THE INNER SMILE VISUALISATION

Please allow about 20 minutes of your time for this lovely exercise.

Make sure that you are not disturbed and make your self-comfortable.

Thank God and the healing angels for helping you achieve divine results with this visualisation.

On the in-breath align yourself with God's divine will and your highest good and highest purpose.

On the out-breath release and let go of all that is not love.

As you carry on breathing, you become aware of a force field of love and light surrounding you.

As you breathe out, all tensions and worries leave your body, draining away into the ground.

When you are ready, grow golden roots from the soles of your feet down through the layers of the earth, where in mid-earth they meet with a pool of emerald-coloured light.

Dip your roots into this wonderful emerald vibration and on the in-breath draw it all the way up into your foot chakras.

Release and let go on the out-breath.

On the next breath, allow this beautiful emerald light to rise up into your base chakra, filling it with this delightful vibration.

Release and let go on the out-breath.

Take another deep breath in and allow the emerald green vibration to rise up further into your sacral chakra flooding it with emerald green light.

Release and let go on the out-breath.

With the next in-breath, bring the emerald light into your solar plexus area.

Release and let go on the out-breath.

When you are ready take another breath in and allow the emerald green light to flow into your heart chakra.

Now your heart centre is filled to overflowing with this magical emerald green vibration.

Release and let go on the out-breath.

Next you become aware of a golden cloud above your head.

A radiant golden beam of light emerges from the cloud and, as you take an in-breath, it flows into your crown chakra, filling it with golden healing light.

Release and let go on the out-breath.

With the next in-breath, allow the golden vibration to flow into your third eye chakra, flooding in with light.

Release and let go on the out-breath.

As you breathe in again, the golden light flows into your throat chakra, filling it with its wonderful vibration.

Release and let go on the out-breath.

When your are ready, take another deep breath in and allow the golden healing vibration to flow into your emerald-light filled heart chakra, where it forms a golden sun at the centre of it.

Release and let go on the out-breath.

Now put your awareness into the golden sun at the centre of your heart chakra.

Take a deep golden breath in and give a beautiful smile, smile with your heart as well as with your mouth and eyes.

As you do this, the golden sun at your centre becomes bigger and brighter.

Give a smile of deep gratitude for all the good things you have got in your life.

Release and let go on the out-breath.

On the next in-breath of golden light allow this smile to spread to the rest of your body.

Smile your golden smile into every organ, into every gland, into every muscle and every bone of your body and see the sun at your heart centre increasing in light.

Release and let go on the out-breath.

When you are ready, take in another deep breath of golden light and from the centre of your, now, large, radiant sun, smile at all your thoughts and your feelings and smile at your glorious present and future.

Release and let go on the out-breath.

On the next in-breath, allow yourself to smile at the world at large visualising love and peace reigning supreme on earth.

Release and let go on the out-breath.

When you are ready, draw your golden roots out of the pool of emerald green light and bring them back up through the layers of the earth, leaving them just a few inches deep in the ground.

Now close down your chakras. Starting with your crown chakra imagine each chakra to be an open lotus flower.

When you are ready see the flower closing its beautiful petals and finally seal it by placing a golden cross, surrounded by a golden circle on top of it.

Repeat all the way down to the base chakra. Become aware of a huge golden bubble made of electric-blue light right in front of you.

When you are ready, step forward into the bubble, which closes around you.

You are now safe and protected for the rest of the day.

Give thanks to God and the healing angels for their love and cooperation with this exercise.

The joy diet

Quite simply, a joy diet means that you are going to allow yourself all the pleasures you have denied yourself for so long.

First enjoy the small stuff on a regular basis:

> **Have time to yourself every day to do nothing.**
>
> **Buy yourself some flowers.**
>
> **Make time to communicate with nature.**
>
> **Go for a walk in the park.**
>
> **Buy yourself a book or a magazine.**

Watch the latest movie in the cinema.

Have a cup of coffee in your favourite coffee bar.

Have your nails done, or for the men, a professional shave.

Treat yourself to a new perfume or aftershave lotion.

Get a new hairstyle and be daring.

Buy the outfit you have been ogling up for the last few weeks.

Then move on to the bigger stuff:

Take the singing lessons you have wanted to take for years.

Join the dance club your feet are aching to get into.

Climb the mountain you have always wanted to conquer.

Build the house of your dreams.

Have the relationship of your dreams.

Travel to wherever your heart takes you.

I am sure as you allow yourself to get into the joy of things your list will grow and grow. Enjoy!

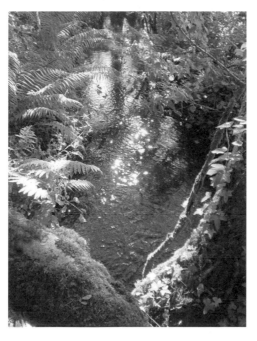

And most of all delight in the joy of being you!

Food for the mind

"Wisdom is the supreme part of happiness."
—Sophocles

The mind thirsts for things to delight in. It looks forward to being nurtured in an uplifting way, reading good books, watching exciting movies and being creative in one way or another.

Most of all, the mind likes to take time off to dream.

It is important to allow the mind to do this, as dreaming is not, as it might seem, a waste of time, but the first step in the act of creativity.

When we take time out in contemplation or meditation, divine sparks of inspiration reach the mind and, if we choose to do so, we can turn these tiny sparks into our dream reality.

For the dream we desire from the depth of our hearts with all our might and passion is the very mission God has intended us to fulfil in this life on earth.

The resonance of joy is equal to the resonance of unconditional love and light.

The happier we are, the more love and light emanates from our being, the more healing will happen all around us.

In our happiest moments our connection to God is the strongest and we will do the greatest service to the world by following our dreams.

We all have dreams; lets bring them forth into a glorious new reality.

"The man who has no imagination has no wings."
— Muhammad Ali

The dream diet

To go on a dream diet you must first and foremost allow yourself the time to dream. If you take the time to go for a walk in nature or for a long drive through glorious countryside, or to sit in the garden or lie in a bath filled with essential oils and rose petals, you will get in touch with your big dream.

The biggest dreams, I have learned, are mostly the ones we have yearned for since childhood so you need to travel back in time and find out what you were daydreaming

Creating with the power of music

"Music is a mediator between spiritual and sensual life."
—Ludwig von Beethoven

Music, glorious music! What would our lives be like without it? Music truly makes the soul sing and the spirit soars; it delights and uplifts. What a wonderful gift it is to hear the little lark singing in the sky and to listen to a Mozart violin concerto, heavenly delights, indeed.

The high vibration of music is able to lift our emotions, mind and spirit out of the daily grind and to soothe and uplift our lives.

The energy of music has a powerful effect on our chakras and energy field, acting as a kind of tuning fork when it hits the auric field. For example, it's great to do the vacuuming to Rock and Roll music because it stimulates the base chakra which gets us going,

The powerful effect of certain music on our mental and emotional bodies has now been proven; it's been dubbed "the Mozart Effect". In a series of experiments, school children were played various works of Mozart while they did their schoolwork; it was found that this music had a calming effect on the children and enhanced their ability to concentrate.

Anyone who composes music does so passionately and it is this creative energy that uplifts us when we listen to such compositions.

Music is a way for the soul to express itself.

When we have an idea or inspiration and we feel passionate about it, then our souls have become involved in the creative process. We can use the power of music to charge our desires with heavenly energy, to enable them to manifest more rapidly.

"Everything has its music.
Everything has genes of God inside."
—Hafiz

CREATING YOUR DREAMS WITH MUSIC VISUALISATION

Concentrate on what you would like to create and do "as if" by imagining that it has already become a reality.

Try to sense what it feels like to have this dream fulfilled. Make the picture and feeling as vivid as possible.

Thank God for giving you this opportunity and feel gratitude filling your heart.

Play the piece of music that makes your "heart sing" the most; then either write your ideas down or sing along with the music having your dream firmly fixed in your heart and mind. (Mozart's violin concerto is playing in the background as I'm writing this.)

Put all your enthusiasm and passion behind this process and let the musical notes be a vehicle for your creation.

Soon your dream will manifest into tangible form for yourself and the world to enjoy!

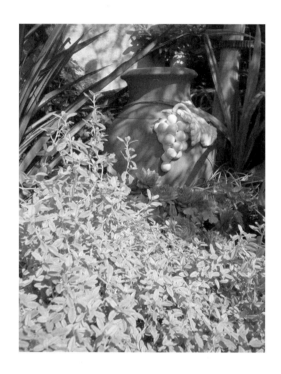

**"What ever you can do or dream you can, begin it.
Boldness has genius, magic and power in it."
— *Johann Wolfgang Goethe***

Food for the emotions

*"It is only with the heart that one can see rightly,
what is essential is invisible to the eye."*
—Antoine de Saint-Exupery

What do our hearts truly yearn for? It is love, love and more love our hearts would like to feel.

The love diet

Give your heart what it truly desires right now! Not by running down the road to find a lover, but by falling in love with yourself.

All the love your heart desires is slumbering within you right now at this present moment.

Like Cinderella it needs to be awakened by a loving kiss.

All your life you've been searching for your prince or princess outside yourself, which has brought much heartache in its wake.

In this story, however, you are both princess and prince, as your soul has been housing within it all the male and female qualities with which you need to complete yourself.

In the divine reality, you are already complete but are not aware of it, causing you to seek outside of yourself for somebody or something to make you complete. The divine law of "like attracts like" states that you attract on the outside experiences which reflect what's going on with you inside. If there's only a tiny flicker of love for yourself in your heart, then anyone you meet will be just like you. Both of you will be unable to express love for each other in the way that you dream of. In order to find unconditional love, we must first be able to give it to ourselves.

Once we are able to fill ourselves with the love and light of our divine self, the need to look for love elsewhere will lessen considerably and might even cease altogether.

Once you feel you've achieved this, you might choose the freedom of a single life, or, now that you are complete within yourself and able to stand on your own two feet spiritually and emotionally, choose to attract a partner who is like you into your life.

As your partner will be truly like you, you are then able to have a wonderful relationship based on unconditional love and mutual respect for each other.

If you are in an existing relationship, then fulfilling your own inner yearning for love will greatly heal and enhance the relationship you do have. As you are now fulfilling your own needs, co-dependency issues, which blight most relationships, will cease to exist and your partnership will be raised to a new loving level.

Remember that it's only love that counts; be loving towards yourself and your partners, friends and family without trying to drag them into your reality. Allow them the freedom to create their own. This is what unconditional love is, allowing ourselves the freedom to be while allowing others to be how they want to be.

Falling in love with yourself is easier said than done, as old thoughts and negative beliefs will creep in, trying to destroy the good work you are doing.

To help you with this ongoing process of learning to love yourself, please work with the following affirmations.

Falling in love with yourself affirmations

I AM THE I AM

I,_____, love myself because I AM.

I,_____, love myself unconditionally for who I am.

I,_____, love myself unconditionally for what I am.

I,_____, love myself unconditionally for what I do.

I,_____, am the proud owner of a loving heart.

I,_____, am a kind person.

I,_____, am a good mother.

I,_____, am a good father.

I,_____, am a good brother.

I,_____, am a good sister.

I,_____, am a good friend.

I,_____, have a nice voice.

I,_____, have lovely eyes.

I,_____, have lovely lips.

I,_____, have a lovely body.

I,_____, am good at _____

I,_____, am good at _____

I,_____, am in love with love.

I hope, that you will have many more items to add to this list.

Read your list out loud as often as possible.

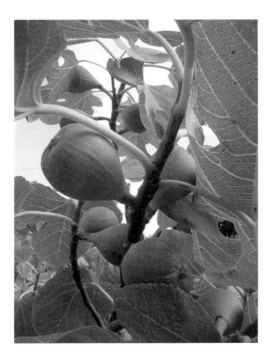

"Love is the music of the universe… just dance!"
—author unknown

Food for the body

"We are what we eat and think. The body becomes what we eat
and the spirit becomes what we think."
—Jesus the Christ

Your glorious body, the temple of your soul, deserves to be treated with special respect and reverence.

It deserves to be fed and watered with tender loving care, taken for walks and regular holidays and made a special fuss of occasionally.

Here is a list of suggestions to make your body a happy one.

Tips for a happy body

- Eat wholesome food, if possible organically grown, vegetarian and GM-free.

- Take plenty of fresh air.

- Spend as much time as possible in nature.

- Have a go at growing your own food.

- Get regular sleep.

- Have power naps.

- Practice relaxation or meditation on a daily basis.

- Do Yoga or other related exercises, to work with your sacred breath.

- Think happy thoughts.

- Say lovely things.

- Feel joyful emotions.

- Practice random acts of kindness often.

- Listen to what your body is trying to tell you.

- Take yourself "lightly".

- Laugh often and heartily.

- Forgive yourself readily.

- Love life.

- Love yourself.

THE IMPORTANCE OF PURE WATER

As 60% of the body is made of water, the quality of the water we drink is of great importance.

Unfortunately tap water contains many harmful chemicals, so it needs to be purified before consumption.

I strongly recommend drinking only mineral or distilled water, if at all possible, and also cooking with it.

Increasing the vibration of the water by blessing it, charging it with crystals or allowing the rays of the sun to infuse it is also beneficial.

Any of these suggestions will bring excellent results and increase the light quotient in the water, which will then increase the amount of light into the body.

Drinking plenty of water during the day is vital. Between six to eight glasses of pure water is the recommended intake for an adult to ensure efficient detoxification and general good maintenance.

Going on a one-day water and fruit fast once a week is a very beneficial way to detoxify the system.

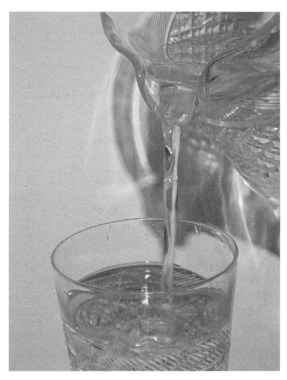

Water is life and there is no life without water!
Thank mother Gaia for this invaluable gift she bestows onto us!

The more light and love in our food the better

L et us just recap and add some positive food affirmations at this point.

- It's not the food which causes us to be over-weight or underweight, but the thoughts we have about the food.

- Our mind creates our reality.

- If we think perfect body-shape, we will have a perfect body-shape, no matter what we eat.

- We need to always eat in moderation and make sure our food is of good quality, physically and energetically.

- The light and love contained within our food is the truly nourishing component of our diet.

- The more light and love that is present in our food, the less we need to eat and the lighter our body will be naturally!

FOOD AFFIRMATIONS

I, _____ , eat what I want, when I want.

I, _____ , am able to eat as much or as little as I like, as my body will tell me what is right for me.

I, _____ , create my own thoughts about which foods are good for me and which ones are not.

I, _____ , love food.

If food is grown with love and tender care in a favourable physical environment, then harvested with respect, delivered to the shops by a nice person and cooked by us while we are in a good mood, then we are on to a winner in the "light stakes".

By what energy is this sequence of events connected?

It is linked by the energy of light and love. If the food grower loved growing the apples, if the fruit pickers had a ball while they were picking them, if the deliveryman was happy to be able to deliver such brilliant produce, then our apple pie will taste like it was made in heaven!

As love equals light, we will end up with a lot of light in our dessert, which is why we will tell the cook, " This is a de-light-full apple pie".

This is, of course a bit of a dream scenario, and doesn't happen too often. However we can, if we want, get our food from local organic growers, or health food stores and cut down on factory-produced food. An apple in the supermarket might look good, but how much light and love does it actually contain? Grown in a far-flung country; picked by underpaid workers, subjected to chemicals to make it keep for a long time, shipped in cold, dark containers; left to ripen; then when it finally arrives in the supermarket, it might be unpacked by a tired, grumpy person in the middle of the night. Every single transaction that happens to this apple leaves an energy imprint behind, which becomes intrinsically part of the fruit.

The frightening thing is that we absorb this negative energy into our energy field the moment we take the first bite.

In scenario number one, the energy imprinted will be lots of love and light; number two is a different story of very mixed energies.

When we eat the apple of scenario number one, we think that this was a delicious apple and feel good after eating it.

However, after consuming the apple of scenario number two, which might just about taste ok, we may not feel too good; in some cases our energy, depending on how sensitive we are, will take a nose-dive.

How to avoid the "bad apples"?

Very simply, when we go shopping for our food we need to listen to our intuition. When we even look at certain foods their appearance does not appeal to us, which really means that their energy is not appealing to us.

In essence, what we consume is the light=life-force of the food. As soon as the food is removed from its source, like the apple from the tree, its life-force starts to diminish; the longer the apple takes to get to the table the less life-force=light is available to us. Many important vitamins, minerals and other healing qualities of our food are lost forever that way.

Remember as well:

- To make sure your food is of good quality, physically and energetically.
- Never buy food because it's cheap. (You'll need far less if you eat light-filled foods.)
- To refrain from micro-waving your food, as this kills the life-force it contains.
- Most of all listen to your body, it will tell you specifically what you need to eat.

Foods that heal

We will benefit from treating ourselves to plenty of fresh fruits and vegetables and also including plenty of pulses, grains and seeds in our diet. Sunflower and pumpkin seeds are an excellent source of protein, a good source of vitamin E and the B vitamins, a good source of fibre and high in unsaturated fats.

To strengthen the immune system, we can add seasonal berries such as raspberries, strawberries, blueberries and cranberries to our diet, as they supply good amounts of vitamin C plus potassium, which has a vital role in maintaining the body's mineral and fluid balance. All berries have antioxidant properties and so help to prevent degenerative diseases.

There follows a list of some "super foods", chosen because of their special abilities to help fight illness and/or promote good health.

Try to include these foods in your diet on a regular basis, unless you are allergic to any of them or have been advised by your doctor to avoid them.

This list doesn't imply that other foods are not good for you, it's just that here I have picked out the ones that are especially beneficial for your health.

SUPER FOODS:

- Asparagus: a good source of vitamin E and a natural diuretic
- Avocado: a very good source of vitamin E and monounsaturated fats, also contains many other vitamins and minerals
- Broad beans: excellent source of fibre plus a range of minerals and vitamins
- Green broccoli: high in fibre, antioxidant vitamins and vitamin C
- Brussels sprouts: are thought to contain natural antiseptic properties
- Savoy cabbage: many vitamins and minerals
- Sweet potato, orange fleshed: rich in beta-carotene, a good source of vitamins E and C
- Butternut squash: rich in carotenoids and good source of vitamins E and C
- Tomatoes: rich in beta-carotene, vitamins C and E, contains lycopene and strong a antioxidant
- Kale: good source of antioxidants and plenty of vitamins C and E
- Spanish onions: contain natural antibiotics and may help to lower blood cholesterol
- Garlic: contains an antioxidant that lowers blood cholesterol and prevents clotting, also contains allicin, which is antibiotic, anti-fungal and possibly antiviral
- Fresh chillies: aid digestion, relieve congestion, contain high level of the painkiller and antioxidant capsaicin, the same as red peppers
- Fresh peas: good source of vitamin C, fibre and many other vitamins
- Red peppers: one of the best sources of vitamin C in vegetables, high in beta-

carotene, contain natural painkiller capsaicin, may be useful against arthritis pain.

- Adzuki beans: low in fat and cholesterol-free, high in protein, fibre, iron and vitamin B with good levels of zinc and other vitamins and minerals

- Chick peas, haricot beans, lentils, soya beans and black-eyed beans have similar properties

- Brown rice: good source of vitamin B, some fibre and low in fat

- Wholemeal pasta: rich in fibre, source of some iron

- Wholemeal flour: lots of fibre and good source of complex carbohydrates

(Please note: many health problems are brought on by wheat/gluten allergies, if in doubt please have an allergy test.)

- Almonds, brazil nuts, cashew nuts and hazelnuts: good amounts of iron, zinc and magnesium

- Sunflower seeds: good source of many minerals

- Mango: best fruit source of antioxidant carotenoids, very rich in fibre, very good source of vitamin E

- Fresh apricots: high in beta-carotene

- Banana: same as apricots plus good source of potassium and manganese

- Eating apple: good vitamin C content depending on variety, contains the flavonoid quercetin which may help lower blood cholesterol

- Blackberries: high amounts of antioxidant vitamin E

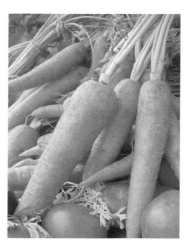

The fresher the food, the more life force is contained within!

Most of us will get cravings for certain foods at certain times, which is perfectly normal; however if we have a balanced diet, these cravings will be few and far between.

If we eat well, the body gets what it needs at the time without plunging into an energy low, which then produces sudden cravings for specific foods.

As our vibratory rate speeds up and more light enters our system, we become more sensitive and naturally veer towards a vegetarian diet.

However, if you feel that eating meat is still important for your general well-being, please be mindful of these factors:

• Animals experience fear before being killed in slaughterhouses and the meat absorbs this vibration of fear. As you eat this meat you absorb this slow, low-frequency energy of fear into your own energy field. If you choose to eat meat try to buy kosher or halal meat where the animal was prayed over and blessed during slaughter.

• As like attracts like, with this fear vibration present in your chakras, an aura of fear will be present and you will now attract more fear towards yourself from the outside world.

• The outcome will be a blocking of the lower chakras, the base, sacral, and to a degree, the solar plexus chakra, as well as the secondary chakras in the soles of the feet. This will hinder the release of the negative energies into mother earth.

Please allow your intuition to guide you as to where to buy meat if you feel you need to eat any and always remember to give thanks to the animal that has sacrificed its life for you.

As I have pointed out blessing our food is a very important practice, as it will channel some of the life-force that was lost in transit from the source to the table back into our food. Also, as it is difficult to avoid microwaved food when eating out, blessing is an excellent way to restore some of the life-force=light value.

Even a simple blessing will give food more energy, but I recommend using either the blessings with golden light or the blessing with silver light.

(Please keep in your mind and heart that blessing meat does not condone either poor animal welfare or slaughter and should not be used as an excuse to keep eating it. However, there are different points-of-view on the subject, and we must each ask ourselves what feels right for us in the matter.)

LIGHT EATING-PLAN SUGGESTIONS

Please find below some examples of how to use the healing and light properties of food for specific purposes.

A one day detox:

The best way to detox for a day is to avoid cooked foods; stick to raw ones, which will have plenty of light in them. Avoid alcohol, tea, coffee, colas and sweets.

Drink plenty of water, at least six to eight glasses over the whole day.

On rising: some hot water with lemon, or water followed by a glass of apple juice

Breakfast: fresh fruit salad with seeds of your choice

Mid-morning: another glass of apple juice

Lunch: large fresh salad, with plenty of grated carrots and celery, lemon juice dressing and nuts of your choice

Mid-afternoon: green tea or another glass of apple juice

Dinner: avocado with lemon juice and sliced tomatoes, seeds of your choice

Bedtime: camomile tea

A day of light eating:

On this day avoid starchy foods and drink plenty of pure water.

Avoid alcohol, tea, coffee, colas and sugar.

On rising: hot water and lemon juice

Breakfast: chopped fresh fruit and a little yofu or natural bio yoghurt, seeds of your choice, (sunflower seeds are recommended)

Mid-morning: apple or fruit of your choice

Lunch: hummus with chopped tomatoes and cucumber

Mid-afternoon: a banana

Dinner: red pepper stuffed with brown rice and herbs, green-leaf salad with olive oil dressing

A day to calm your nerves:

On this day please avoid anything containing caffeine, such as tea, coffee, colas, cocoas and chocolate.

On rising: camomile tea

Breakfast: brown rice pudding, topped with a kiwi and chopped almonds

Mid-morning: two oranges or other citrus fruits

Lunch: lentil and broad bean salad on a bed of green leaves with seeds of your choice

Mid-afternoon: apricot bar

Dinner: nut loaf with steamed broccoli

Bedtime: camomile tea

A day to cheer you up:

On this day please avoid tea, coffee or colas and alcohol.

On rising: hot water with lemon juice

Breakfast: mango with yofu or natural bio yoghurt

Mid-morning: fruit smoothy made with kiwis and banana

Lunch: fresh green pea soup with a dollop of natural crème fraiche and sesame seeds

Mid-afternoon: apricot and date flapjack

Dinner: Butternut squash filled with lentils and herbs with green leaf salad, olive oil dressing

Bedtime: apple

A day to strengthen your immune system:

For this day please cut down on sugar and caffeine and avoid animal fats and alcohol; drink plenty of water and herbal teas.

On rising: hot water with lemon juice

Breakfast: sugar-free muesli with fresh chopped fruits, mainly citrus fruits and nuts and seeds of your choice

Mid-morning: two kiwi fruits

Lunch: sweet potato salad with fresh spinach leaves, olive oil dressing and seeds of your choice, slice of rye bread

Mid-afternoon: fresh berries with a little yofu or natural bio yoghurt

Dinner: vegetable fried rice with broccoli, red peppers and plenty of carrots, sesame and other seeds of your choice

Bedtime: sage or echinacea tea

A day to get your appetite back:

Please avoid alcohol.

On rising: hot water with lemon juice

Breakfast: banana porridge with pumpkin seeds

Mid-morning: fruit smoothy made with mango, kiwi and strawberries

Lunch: baked sweet potato (orange fleshed) with red pepper and sesame salad

Mid-afternoon: fresh strawberries with organic cream

Dinner: nut-cutlets with steamed carrots and broccoli

I sincerely hope that the these suggestions will give you food for thought on how to improve your diet and, most of all, to enjoy your food.

Ultimately the hunger we feel is symbolic for the spiritual hunger we feel for God…and if we refuse to eat, we refuse the love God is waiting to bestow onto us…

Just follow your heart and you will have the best diet there is!

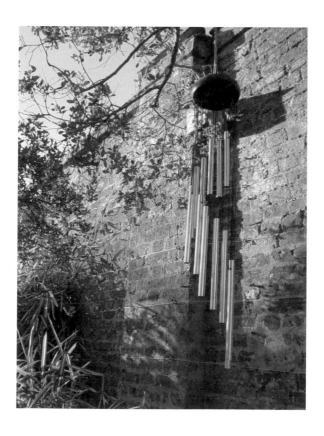

Part 8:
Light Diet Recipes

The following recipes are based on the super foods listed earlier. Do use as many fresh ingredients as possible and buy organic if you can.

For easy, speedy preparation, measurements are given in cups and grams or millilitres for liquid measures. Using cups is really very convenient, if you don't have a set of real measuring cups use a tea cup and just keep using the same cup for half or quarter cups.

Salads

ALFALFA SPROUTS AND AVOCADO SALAD

In this salad, the avocados are stuffed with healthy alfalfa sprouts.

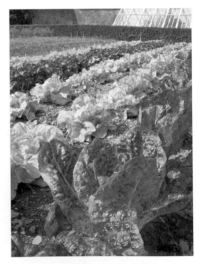

4 avocados (allow 1 avocado per person) cut in half lengthwise and de-stoned

Juice of ½ lemon or lime, freshly squeezed

4 tablespoons mayonnaise

2 tablespoons plain, live yoghurt

1 tablespoon coarse grain french mustard

alfalfa sprouts

green salad

cherry tomatoes to garnish

Cover serving plate generously with the green salad. Sprinkle the exposed surface of the avocado halves with the lemon or lime juice. You may leave the avocado in its shell. Mound the alfalfa sprouts into the cavity left by the stone and place on the serving plate. Combine the mayonnaise, yoghurt and mustard to make a dressing. Spoon dressing over the avocados and garnish with cherry tomatoes. Serves 4.

THREE BEAN SALAD

A filling salad, which could be served as a light lunch.

2 cups (280g) of cooked mixed beans (such as adzuki, haricot or black eyed beans)

2 stalks of celery, chopped

up to 1 cup (140g) raw, fresh red onions, chopped

2 free range eggs, hard boiled and chopped (optional)

2 tablespoons organic olive oil

2 tablespoons balsamic vinegar

lemon wedge

sea salt to taste

freshly ground pepper to taste

Combine all the above ingredients and let the salad sit for an hour to allow the flavours to develop fully. Serves 4.

SWEET POTATO SALAD

This salad is a delicious alternative to ordinary potato salad.

3 cups (450g) sweet potatoes, steamed and sliced

¾ cup (80g) mayonnaise

¼ cup (30g) plain, live yoghurt

1½ tablespoons fresh lemon juice

¼ teaspoon sea salt

freshly ground pepper to taste

¼ cup (30g) chopped fresh chillies or scallions/spring onions

¼ cup (30g) chopped sweet red pepper

paprika to season

The cooked potatoes can be at room temperature or chilled. Combine mayonnaise, yoghurt, lemon juice, salt and pepper to make a smooth dressing. Add scallions, sweet peppers and potatoes, stir gently to coat well without breaking up potatoes. Sprinkle with paprika. Serves 4.

Soups

CHICKPEA AND CARROT PUREE

The flavours of this soup meld together beautifully, offering a hint of garlic and mint. Adding yoghurt enhances both the flavour and the food value of the soup.

1½ cups (225g) cooked chickpeas, drained
3 cups (450g) carrots, diced
2 cloves garlic, crushed
½ cup (65g) red onions, chopped
4 cups (920ml) bean-liquid, water or vegetable stock
1½ teaspoons dried mint
1 tablespoon freshly squeezed lime or lemon juice
sea salt
freshly ground pepper
fresh mint leaves to garnish (optional)
plain, live yoghurt (the Greek version lends itself very well to this dish)

Place chickpeas, carrots and liquid in a pot and bring to the boil. Cover and simmer until carrots are tender enough to puree, about 20 minutes. Puree using either a blender or a food processor and return to the pot. Add dried mint, lemon juice, salt and freshly milled pepper to taste. Simmer for 5 minutes over a low heat. Serve sprinkled with freshly chopped mint (optional) and add yoghurt to each bowl at the table. Serves 4.

BROCCOLI AND MACARONI SOUP

This hearty soup could be served as a very satisfying lunch.

1 tablespoon olive oil
1 clove garlic, chopped
4 cups (920ml) tomato puree (can be made from fresh or tinned tomatoes)
1 teaspoon sea salt
freshly ground pepper to taste
4 cups (400g) chopped broccoli
1 cup (100g) small whole-wheat pasta shells or macaroni
¼ cup (25g) grated parmesan cheese

Heat the olive oil in a pot and sauté garlic until lightly coloured. Add the tomato puree season with salt and pepper to taste and bring to the boil. Add the broccoli cover pot and simmer for 10 minutes. Add the pasta and simmer for a further 10 minutes or until the pasta and broccoli are tender. Serve sprinkled with cheese. Serves 4.

Fresh Homemade Tomato Soup

This homemade soup is well worth the extra effort and will delight your fellow diners.

2 tablespoons butter
1 medium onion, chopped
1 clove garlic, chopped
1 carrot, chopped
1 stalk celery, chopped
4 cups (675g) chopped tomatoes (if you prefer to make the soup without the tomato skins blanch the tomatoesin boiling water and peel)
3 cups (460ml) spring water
1 tablespoon fresh basil (or, if not available, 1 teaspoon dried)
1 teaspoon sea salt
½ teaspoon of brown sugar
2 teaspoons tomato paste (if soup is made from winter tomatoes or tinned tomatoes)
crème fraiche as a garnish (optional)

Melt the butter in a pot and sauté the garlic, onion, carrot and celery for 5 minutes, until the onion is transparent. Add tomatoes and simmer for 10 minutes, mashing them with a wooden spoon until soft and pulpy. Now add water and seasonings and bring to the boil. Simmer uncovered for 20 minutes if the soup is to be pureed, for 30 minutes if it is not. Puree if desired in a blender or food processor. Reheat before serving and add a spoonful of crème fraiche to each bowl to garnish. Serves 4.

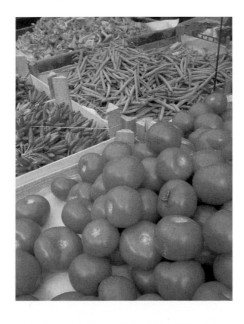

Main Courses

PAELLA

A lovely dish without meat.

>   *3 tablespoons olive oil*
>
>   *1 large onion, chopped*
>
>   *½ tablespoon chopped garlic*
>
>   *1 medium sweet red pepper, chopped*
>
>   *1½ cups (225g) uncooked long grain brown rice*
>
>   *3 cups (690ml) diluted tomato juice (liquid from canned tomatoes or tomato juice diluted with an equal amount of water)*
>
>   *1 teaspoon sea salt*
>
>   *1 teaspoon saffron*
>
>   *1 cup (100g) green peas*
>
>   *2 cups (200g) cooked chick peas or haricot, soya, black eyed or adzuki beans or a mixture of them*
>
>   *2 large fresh artichokes or 1 can (400g)*
>
>   *1 red chilli, chopped*

Heat the oil in a pan and sauté onion, garlic, sweet pepper and rice for about 5 minutes until the rice begins to colour. Add the diluted tomato juice, salt and saffron. Bring to the boil, cover and cook over a low heat for 15 minutes. Meanwhile prepare the artichokes by cutting into medium sized pieces. Add the artichokes together with the peas and beans to the rice and cook, covered, for another 30 minutes or until rice is tender. Garnish with fresh chilli. Serves 4.

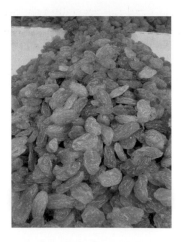

VEGETABLE GOULASH

A firm winter favourite, making good use of the fresh vegetables you happen to have in store.

2 large onions

2 cloves garlic, finely chopped

1 large red or orange pepper

500g potatoes

500g carrots or alternatively 250g carrots and 250g parsnips

375g cabbage (savoy cabbage if you can get it)

1½ tablespoons sunflower oil

2 tablespoons mild paprika

generous pinch cayenne pepper (optional)

2 tablespoons balsamic vinegar

460ml spring water

1½ teaspoons sea salt

100g sour cream or crème fraiche

1 tablespoon of white flour

Wash the root vegetables and cut into approximately 1 inch chunks (peel only if strictly necessary as many of the vitamins and minerals are to be found in the outer layers). Heat oil in a pot and sauté the garlic, onions, peppers and root vegetables for a few minutes to soften. Add the paprika and cayenne pepper and stir thoroughly. Then add the balsamic vinegar, stir and allow it to "cook off". Now add the cabbage, water and salt. Bring to the boil and simmer over a low heat until the vegetables are quite tender, approximately 40 minutes. Mix the sour cream or crème fraiche with the flour, to prevent it curdling and then stir into the goulash.

Simple garlic bread is a great accompaniment to this dish. Serves 4.

STUFFED PEPPERS ITALIAN STYLE

A simple but delicious way to cook stuffed peppers on top of the stove.

4 medium red (or orange) peppers

2 cups (200g) ricotta cheese

1 cup (100g) shredded mozzarella cheese

2 tablespoons grated parmesan cheese

½ teaspoon oregano

1 free-range egg

freshly milled pepper and sea salt to taste

2 cups (460ml) of Italian style tomato sauce well flavoured with garlic, basil and oregano

(This is easily made in a blender or food processor using tinned tomatoes and the seasonings)

Cut the peppers in half through the stem, remove the seeds and any thick inside ribs. Mix the three cheeses with the egg and oregano, adding salt and pepper to taste. Fill pepper halves. Heat tomato sauce in a pan large enough to hold your four stuffed peppers in a single layer and simmer for about 10 minutes to allow the flavours of the herbs to develop. Arrange the peppers stuffing side up in the sauce, cover and simmer over a low heat for about 20 minutes until the peppers are tender but still a little crisp. Spoon tomato sauce over peppers when serving. Accompany with brown rice or a simple leaf salad. Serves 4.

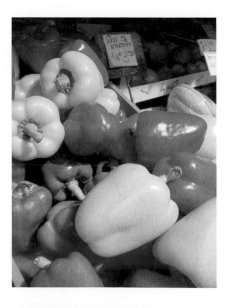

Desserts

EXOTIC BANANA CREAM

This is a creamy frozen fruit dessert, as nice as ice cream, but with much less fat and sugar.

1 ripe banana
1 tablespoon lemon or lime juice fresh
1½ tablespoons honey
1 cup (100g) ricotta cheese

Puree the banana with the lemon juice and honey in a blender or food processor. Add the ricotta and blend until smooth and light. Pour into a container and freeze. Serve when firm but not quite hard. Serves 4.

FRUIT CRUMBLE

You may use a variety of fruits for this dish, such as apples (as in this recipe), blackberries, apricots or blueberries.

3 medium apples cut into bite size pieces
2 tablespoons raisins
½ teaspoon cinnamon
¾ cup (75g) oats
¼ cup (25g) whole-wheat flour
pinch sea salt
2 tablespoons sunflower oil
½ cup apple juice
3 tablespoons honey

Preheat oven to 180°C. Mix together apples, raisins and cinnamon in an oiled, shallow baking dish. Place the oats, flour and salt in a mixing bowl, add the oil and mix until crumbly. Cover apples with crumble topping. Combine the apple juice with the honey, heating it gently if necessary to blend. Pour evenly over the crumble topping. Bake for about 45 minutes and serve topped with yoghurt. Serves 4.

RICE PUDDING WITH APRICOTS

You may substitute raisins for the apricots in this yummy pudding.

> *2 cups (160g) cooked brown rice*
> *2 free range eggs lightly beaten*
> *2 cups (460ml) milk*
> *6 tablespoons honey*
> *½ teaspoon cinnamon*
> *½ teaspoon nutmeg, freshly grated if possible*
> *½ cup (50g) dried apricots, chopped*
> *½ teaspoon vanilla extract*

Place all ingredients except vanilla in a saucepan. Cook over low heat stirring constantly until the mixture thickens. Do not allow to boil. This will take approximately 15 to 20 minutes. Finally stir in vanilla.

Pour pudding into individual dishes, serve either warm or chilled. Serves 4.

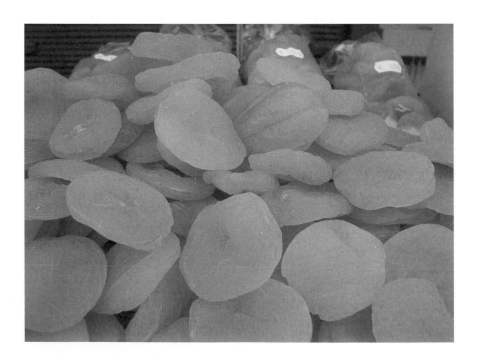

Sprouting

A wonderful, easy way to increase your intake of fresh vitamins and minerals at your leisure is to sprout your own. There are several glass-sprouters on the market, which are inexpensive and easy to use. However you may make your own makeshift sprouter by just using an ordinary glass jar.

THE PROCESS OF SPROUTING:

- Rinse the glass jar with cold water
- Do the same with the seedlings you are about to sprout
- Place 2 – 4 tablespoons of seeds into the jar
- Allow to soak (for soaking time, see preparation information)
- Rinse and allow water to drain away
- Place your jar in a light, warm position, but not into direct sunlight
- Rinse daily, see preparation information
- Harvesting can be done within a few days

SOME OF THE SEEDS AND BEANS YOU CAN SPROUT ARE:

- Alfalfa
- Fenugreek
- Lentils
- Mung bean
- Little radish
- French turnip
- Wheat

SOME FAVOURITES AND HOW TO BEST SPROUT THEM:

Alfalfa sprouts: contain among other things vitamins A, B2, C, D and niacin as well as a host of minerals, such as iron, magnesium, all 8 essential amino acids, protein, chlorophyll and fibre.

Preparation: Use 2 to 4 tablespoons per glass jar, soak for 4 hours and rinse once a day. Keep the sprouts at a temperature of between 18-22°C for about 6-8 days.

Fenugreek sprouts: contain among other things vitamins A, B1, B2, B5, and D, iron, phosphorus and niacin.

Preparation: Use 2 to 4 tablespoons per glass jar, soak for 5 hours and rinse twice a day. Keep the sprouts at a temperature of between 18-22°C for 2-3 days.

Mung bean sprouts: contain among other things, vitamins A, B1, B2, B3, B6 and C, iron, potassium, calcium, magnesium and phosphorus.

Preparation: Use 2 to 4 tablespoons per glass jar, soak for 12 hours and rinse twice a day. Keep the sprouts at a temperature of between 18-22°C for 4-5 days.

Treat yourself to a portion of fresh sprouts a day, either as a salad or topping on baked potatoes or sandwiches and see your energy levels increase!

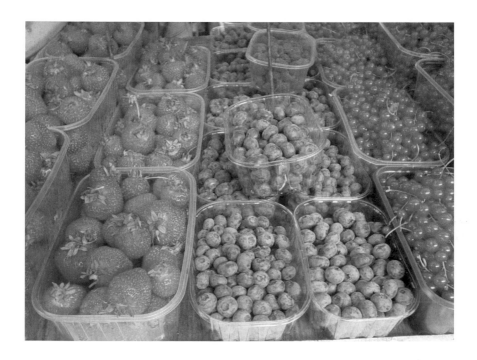

Juicing

Fresh juices are not only a vital part of any detox programme, but also provide vital energy if taken on a regular basis.

Juices are best prepared using a juicer and must be consumed immediately, in order not to loose the important vitamins and minerals, which are only present in the fresh produce.

LIST OF FRUITS AND VEGETABLES YOU CAN JUICE:

Fruits: Apples, Pears, Bananas, Melons, Peaches, Nectarines, Apricots, Grapefruit, Oranges, Lemons, Limes, Mangoes, Papapayas, Pineapples, Grapes, Strawberries.

Vegetables: Carrots, Beetroot, Tomatoes, Lettuce, Cabbage, Watercress, Fennel Bulb, Spinach, Cucumber.

This list is just suggestions in order to inspire you to use your imagination for many more juicing ideas.

HERE ARE SOME SUGGESTIONS TO GET YOU JUICING:

Apple Mix: Apple, grapes and a dash of lime.

Grapefruit Mix: Grapefruit, orange and a little lemon juice.

Tropical Mix: Mango, pineapple and a dash of lime.

Starwberry Mix: Starwberries and apricots.

Carrot Mix: Carrots, beetroot, grapes and a little fesh ginger.

Pick-me-up Mix: Tomatoes, cucumber, garlic, fresh parsley, dash of lemon juice.

Detox Mix: Watercress, grapes, apple and a little fresh lime juice.

Classic Mix: Orange, apple an carrots.

Your physical health can greatly benefit from a juice day once a week. This will give your bowels a rest, allowing toxins to leave your system, leaving you fresh and rejuvinated the next day.

Give it a try!

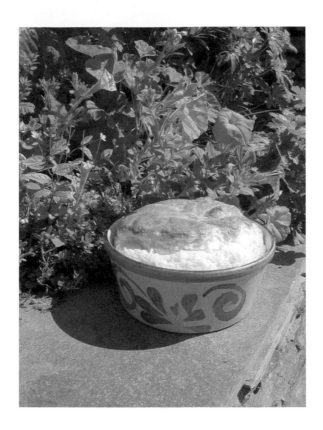

"There are many paths to enlightenment.
Be sure to take one with a heart."
—*Lao Tzu*

Introducing the forever-light technique

The forever-light technique consists of a series of simple but vital affirmations encapsulating the contents of this book.

It is designed for fast and efficient use and takes only a few minutes to carry out. However, it does take a little time to memorise. You might want to type it out and hang it on your bedroom or bathroom wall for a few days until you know its contents by heart.

Please use it every day, preferably in the morning, for maximum success and benefit.

The forever-light technique

Upon opening your eyes:

Mentally align yourself with God's divine will and the highest purpose for yourself and all sentient beings on this planet.

Ask for God's blessings for your day and thank Him for giving you the best day of your life.

Thank your guardian angels, for looking after you, day and night.

As you are getting up:

Affirm to yourself: I accept myself as I am.

I am doing the best I can today.

Whatever happens today, I am free to choose again.

As you get into the shower:

Affirm to yourself: I release all that is not love.

I let go and let God

As you get dressed:

Visualise the perfect divine you standing in front of you giving you a lovely smile.

Walk forward and merge with the perfect divine you.

Look out through your divine eyes into the world.

And know that you are within God and God is within you, you are ONE!

Have the best day of your life!

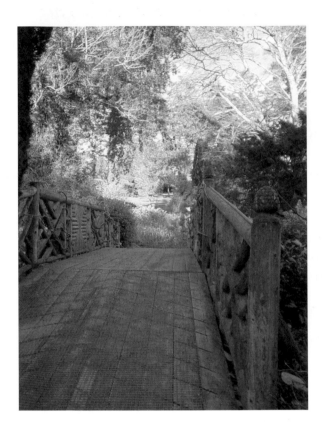

This, my dear soul brothers and soul sisters, is my humble offering to you.

I pray that the book has helped a little on your journey, that it has provided you with insight and given you the strength and courage to be your true, divine, glorious self.

I am delighted that I was given the opportunity to accompany you a little way along the path to love.

May you walk safely in the light.
With heartfelt blessings,

Glossary of Spiritual Terms:

ANGELS: benevolent beings of light and messengers of God dedicated to the enlightenment of humankind

ARCHANGELS: a higher order of the angelic kingdom

AURA: energy field surrounding all life forms

BLOCKAGE: a negative mental or emotional pattern stopping the natural flow of the life force

CHANNELLING: allowing higher energies to flow through us for healing, guidance or inspiration

CHAKRAS: energy centres within the aura

CLEANSING: the act of removing negative energy from our bodies, from other people or objects or locations, by utilising positive intent

DIVINE POWER: the life force, the source of all things, the pure energy which exists within the divine

ELEMENTALS: beings who govern the spirit realm of the elements of earth, fire, water, air and the fifth element, ether

GAIA: the Greek name of the earth mother goddess; also the theory that planet earth is a self-regulating, conscious organism

GOD: the essence behind the form; the source of all there is, incarnate in all: humans, animals, plants and minerals

GROUNDING: energy process that allows the body to connect to the earth

GUIDES: discarnate beings of light who assist human kind in their quest for enlightenment

GUIDED IMAGERY/VISUALISATION: a "mind over matter" technique of imagining positive images to promote mental, emotional, physical and spiritual well-being

HEALING: a conscious channelling of divine energy for ourselves either "hands on" or projected distantly, when it is known as DISTANT HEALING

HIGHER SELF: highest, wisest, all-knowing part of the self; the divine personal aspect of the mind carrying our divine potential or blueprint

INCARNATION: literary means "enfleshment"; the soul inhabits a physical body by taking birth on the earth plane

INNER CHILD: part of the adult self that has not matured emotionally or mentally

KARMA: Hindu and Buddhist belief based on the law of cause and effect, stating that thoughts and deeds, if not balanced out over one lifetime, will be carried forward into the next one, so binding us to "the wheel of karma"

LIGHT: finest universal substance

LOWER SELF/EGO SELF: the "little self" which identifies with the conditioned desires and needs of the lower nature of humanity

MEDITATION: literally a state of "no mind", also a term used for the process for getting into such a state via contemplation, visualisation and guided imagery, etc.

REINCARNATION/REBIRTH: the belief that the soul incarnates into different bodies throughout many lifetimes in order to learn, grow and rediscover its true origin, namely that it is God

SELF-REALIZATION/SELF-ILLUMINATION/ENLIGHTENMENT: synonyms for GOD REALISATION and the personal, conscious recognition of our divinity

SENTIENT: endowed with feeling, sensory perception and consciousness

SOUL: the divine personal aspect of the heart, carrying our life's purpose

SOURCE: divine essence

UNCONDITIONAL LOVE: highest universal vibration, pure love without condition on a human level

UNIVERSAL ENERGY: another term for God, the energy underlying and infusing all there is

Recommended Reading

SPIRITUAL AND PERSONAL SELF DEVELOPMENT:

Bailey, Alice A., *Education in the New Age*, Lucis Press, 1971.

Bailey, Alice A., *Glamour: World Problem*, Lucis Press, 1995.

Bays, Brandon, *The Journey*, Harper-Collins, 1999.

Berg, Michael, *Becoming God*, Kabbalah Publishing, 2004.

Brennan, Barbara A., *Light Emerging: The Journey of Personal Healing*, Bantam, 1993.

Gardener, Mike and Barbara Gardener, *Sathya Sai Baba and You: Practical Spirituality*, Wisdom Works Press, 1991.

Al Haqquani, Sheikh Nazim, *Defending Truth*, Zero Publications, 1997.

Al Haqquani, Sheikh Nazim, *Star from Heaven,* Zero Publications, 1996.

Hay, Louise L., *You Can Heal Your Life*, Full Circle Publishing 2003.

His Holiness the Dalai Lama, *The Art of Happiness,* Penguin, 1998.

His Holiness the Dalai Lama, *Advice on Dying And Living a Better Life*, Atria, 2002.

Knapp, Stephen, *Secret Teachings of the Vedas*, The World Relief Network, 1990.

Krystal, Phyllis, *Cutting the Ties that Bind*, Weiser, 1994.

Mafi, Maryam and Azima Melita Kolin, *Rumi: Gardens of the Beloved*, Element, 2004.

Meyer, Y. Marvin, The Secret Teachings of Jesus: Four Gnostic Gospels, Random House, 1986.

Myss, Caroline, *Anatomy of the Spirit,* Three Rivers Press, 1997.

Myss, Caroline, *Why People Don't Heal and How They Can*, Three Rivers Press, 1998.

Satchidananda, Sri Swami, *The Yoga Sutras of Patanjali*, Integral Yoga Publications, 1984.

Shah, Ali Ikba, *Muhammed: The Prophet*, Tractus books, 1997.

Thich Nhat Hanh, *The Heart of the Buddha's Teaching: Transform suffering into peace, joy and liberation*, Rider, 1999.

Thurman, Robert A. F. (Translator) and H.H. the Dalai Lama (Foreword), *The Tibetan Book Of the Dead: Liberation through Understanding in the Between*, Harper Collins, 1993.

Tolle, Eckhart, *The Power of Now,* New World Library, 1999.

Walsh, Neale Donald, *Conversations with God*, Putnam Publishing Group, 1996.

White Eagle, *Gentle Brother: The Power of Love in Your Life*, White Eagle Publishing Trust, 1968.

White Eagle, *Heal Thyself,* White Eagle Publishing Trust, 1999.

Yogananda, Paramahansa, *Where There Is Light,* Self Realization Fellowship, 1989.

Yogananda, Paramahansa, *Scientific Healing Affirmations*, Self Realization Fellowship, 1958.

THE CHAKRAS AND THE AURIC FIELD:

Brennan, Barbara Ann, *Hands of Light, A Guide to Healing Through the Human Energy Field*, Bantam, 1998.

Johari, Harish, Chakras, *Energy Centres of Transformation*, Diederichs, 2001.

Leadbeater, Charles W., *The Chakras*, Quest Books 1972.

SPIRITUAL HEALING:

Angelo, Jack, *Spiritual Healing, Energy Medicine For Today*, Element, 1991.

Bek, Lilla and Philippa Pullar, *The Seven Levels of Healing*, Rider, 1986.

Bradford, Michael, *Hands-On Spiritual Healing*, Findhorn Press, 1994

Brofman, Martin, *Anything Can Be Healed*, Findhorn Press, 2003.

Edwards, Harry, (the founder of the National Federation of Spiritual Healers, England), *The Power of Spiritual Healing*, Jenkins.

Furlong, David, *The Healer Within*, Piatkus, 2000.

MEDITATION:

Caddy, Eileen, *Opening Doors Within*, Findhorn Press, 1987.

Caddy, Eileen, *The Living Word*, Findhorn Press, 1977.

Harrison, Eric, *How Meditation Heals*, Piatkus, 2000.

Main, Darren John, *The Findhorn Book of Meditation*, Findhorn Press, 2003.

Trungpa, Chogyam, *Meditation in Action*, Shambala, 2004.

ANGELS:

Cooper, Diana, *A Little Light on Angels*, Findhorn Press, 1996.

Lawson, David, *A Company of Angels*, Findhorn Press, 1998.

Virtue, Doreen, *Healing with the Angels*, Hay House, 1999.

EARTH HEALING:

Lovelock, James, *Gaia: A New Look at Life on Earth*, Oxford University Press, 2000.

Stowe, John R., *The Findhorn Book of Connecting with Nature*, Findhorn Press, 2003.

Pogacnik, Marko, *Christ Power Earth Goddess: A Fifth Gospel*, Findhorn Press, 1997.

Pogacnik, Marko, *Earth Changes Human Destiny: Coping and Attuning with the Help of the Revelation of St. John*, Findhorn Press, 2000.

Pogacnik, Marko, *The Daughter of Gaia: Rebirth of the Divine Feminine*, Findhorn Press, 2001.

Pogacnik, Marko, *Healing the Heart of the Earth: Restoring the Subtle Levels of Life*, Findhorn Press, 1998.

Pogacnik, Marko, *Nature Spirits and Elemental Beings: Working with the Intelligence in Nature*, Findhorn Press, 1996.

Roads, Michael J., *Talking with Nature*, New World Library 2003.

Roads, Michael J., *Journey into Nature, a Spiritual Adventure*, H.J. Kramer, 1990.

Stowe, John R., *Earth Spirit Warrior*, Findhorn Press, 2002.

REBIRTHING:

Orr, Leonard and Sondra Ray, *Rebirthing in the New Age*, Celestial Arts, 1983.

KINESIOLOGY:

Eden, Donna and David Feinstein, *Energy Medicine*, Putnam Publishing Group, 2000.

Levy, Susan L. et 'al', *Your Body Can Talk: How to Use Simple Muscle Testing to Learn What Your Body Knows and Needs*, Hohm Press, 1996.

EATING DISORDERS:

Cooper, Peter and Christopher Fairburn, *Bulimia Nervosa and Binge-eating: A Guide to Recovery*, New York University Press, 1997.

Danowski, Debbie and Pedro Lazaro, *Why Can't I Stop Eating? : Recognizing, Understanding and Overcoming Food Addiction*, Hazelden Publishing & Educational Services, 2000

Treasure, Janet, *Breaking free from Anorexia Nervosa: A Survival Guide for Families, Friends and Sufferers*, Psychology Press, 1997.

PAST LIVES:

Weiss, Brian C., *Through Time into Healing*, Fireside, 1993.

Woolger, Roger J., *Healing Your Past Lives,* Sounds True, 2004.

INNER CHILD WORK:

Bradshaw, John, *Homecoming: Reclaiming and Championing Your Inner Child*, Bartram, 1992.

CHILDHOOD ABUSE:

Adamson, Liz, *Overcoming Sexual and Childhood Abuse*, Diviniti Publishing Ltd., 2004.

HYPNOTHERAPY AND REGRESSIONS:

McKenna, Paul, *Change Your life in Seven Days*, Harmony, 2005.

Newton, Michael, *Life Between Lives: Hypnotherapy for Spiritual Regression*, Llewellyn, 2004.

SPIRITUAL NUTRITION:

Cousens, Gabriel, *Spiritual Nutrition and the Rainbow Diet*, North Cassandra Press, 1987.

Virtue Doreen et.al., *Eating in the Light: Making the Switch to Vegetarianism on Your Spiritual Path*, Hay House, 2001.

Gabrielle Chavez, *The Raw Food Diet*, Findhorn Press 2005

NUTRITION:

Emoto, Masaru, *Hidden Messages in Water*, Beyond Words Publishing, 2004.

Holford Patrick, *New Optimum Nutrition Bible*, Crossing Press, 2005.

Mosaraf, Ali, *Dr. Ali's Nutrition Bible*, Vermilion, 2004.

Advice and help pages

TELEPHONE LINES FOR HELP IN THE UK:

Samaritans: 0845 790 9090
24h – If you are in a crisis and need to talk

Sane Line: 0845 767 8000
Emotional Support & Info, noon to 2am

No Panic: 0808 808 0545
National Help line for phobias and anxiety attacks

Cruse: 0870 167 1677
Deals with bereavement

UK National Drugs Helpline: 080 077 6600
Offers free confidential 24h advice

Women's Aid: 0808 2000 247
National domestic violence helpline

Childline: 0800 1111
24h free helpline for children and young people

NAPAC: 0800 085 3330
National Association for People Abused in Childhood

Everyman helpline: 020 7737 6747
Confidential Counselling for men experiencing violence

Medical Advisory Service: 020 8994 9874
6-9pm, advice on health and medical matters

Drink Line: 0800 917 8282

Ash: 0800 00 22 00
smoking quit line

ADVICE AND HELP ON THE WEB IN THE UK:

Childhood abuse:

www,napac.org.uk

NAPAC - National Association for People Abused in Childhood

www.siari.co.uk.

SIARI – Self-injury & Related Issues, NSPCC initiative working with survivors of childhood sexual abuse

www.survivorsuk.co.uk

Help for men who have been sexually abused or raped

www.survivors.org.uk

On-line self-help, support and info group for adult survivors of childhood abuse

Counselling and Psychotherapy:

www.bacp.co.uk

BACP – British Association for Counselling and Psychotherapy

www.counsellingServices.co.uk

www.cccs.co.uk

CCCS - charity providing free counselling

www.onlinecounselling.co.uk

On-line counselling service

Eating disorders:

www.eating-disorders.org.uk

National Centre for Eating Disorders UK – info on treatment, network of specialised counsellors, also telephone-treatment and free assessment

General abuse:

www.womensaid.org.uk

Women's aid – key national charity in UK for woman and children experiencing physical, sexual or emotional abuse in their homes

www.childline.org.uk

Childline, free and confidential help-line for children and young adults

www.recovery.org.uk

Alcohol, drug abuse help

Hypnotherapy:

www.hypnotherapists.org.uk

National Council for Hypnotherapy

www.formative.pwp.blueyonder.co.uk

Psychotherapy and Hypnotherapy Counselling Services

www.hypnotheraph-online.co.uk

Provides hypnotherapy online

www.hypnosis-guide.com

Provides general information

Rebirthing:

www.holisticguide.net/ebirthingorg.html

Rebirthing Organisations in the UK and Holistic Health guide

Reiki Healing:

www.reikifed.co.uk

UK Reiki Federation – gives info on training and guidance on Reiki issues.

www.reikiassociation.org.uk

UK Reiki Association – info on Reiki training and other issues.

Spiritual Healing:

www.holisticguide.net/healingorg.html

Healing organisations in the UK

www.bahahealing.co.uk

BAHA – British Alliance of Healing Organisations

www.nfsh.org.uk

NFSH – National Federation of Spiritual Healers

For information on healing and healer training, ring the Referral Line: 0845 1232767

www.harryedwards.org.uk

Harry Edwards, founder of the NFSH Spiritual Healing Sanctuary

ALSO BY ELISABETH CONSTANTINE

The Light Diet Meditations CD —*the ideal companion to this book!*—

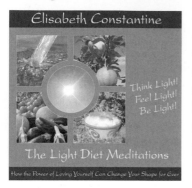

Let Elisabeth guide you through the *Forever Light Diet Plan*. This plan consists of 9 steps to promote right thinking and takes the form of guided visualisations, colour breathing and energy-work. From attunement to your higher, divine self, this CD guides you into the light of your true, happy, fulfilled self. Suitable both for the new meditator as well as those more advanced on the path of meditation.

1-84409-045-0

Light Meditations for a Year:

A Book of Contemplations, Guided Meditations and Positive Affirmations for Every Day of the Year

You are a spiritual being having a physical experience in your body. You yearn for self-illumination, to truly find yourself and your purpose in life. You are a "spiritual work in process." If this is true of you, then the daily contemplations, meditations and affirmations in this book will be welcome companions on your journey of personal transformation, discovery and inner knowledge.

400 pages paperback with black & white photographs

1-84409-038-8

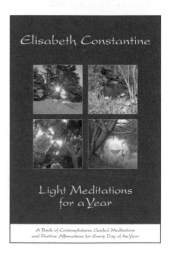

All available from your local bookshop,
or directly from www.findhornpress.com

For up-to-date information on Elisabeth Constantine's work and schedule,
please visit www.light-meditations.com

ALSO BY ELISABETH CONSTANTINE

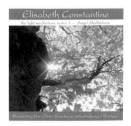

For both the experienced meditator and the beginner alike, here are three invaluable CDs. Tools for learning how to be still and go inside to work on important life issues, or help in going deeper and contacting the higher beings to aid and support your transformation into light, each of these Cds can provide all the support and inspiration you will need.

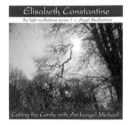

CD1 "Manifesting Your Sacred Inner Sanctuary with Archangel Raphael" will help you create that peaceful place inside yourself where you can take your challenges, big and small, where you can retreat and allow the silence to surround and support you.

CD2 "Cutting the Cords, with Archangel Michael". We all have negative situations and relationships dragging us down, keeping us from living a totally joyful life. This CD will help you release all these no longer needed experiences, gracefully and lovingly.

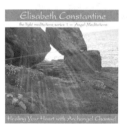

CD3 "Healing you Heart with Archangel Chamuel" will lead you gently into healing all pain and hurt from the past into a free and light filled future. Allow the Archangels to be your friends and allies in your search for your spiritual roots.

- Manifesting Your Inner Sanctuary with Archangel Raphael   1-84409-039-6
- Cutting the Cords, with Archangel Michael   1-84409-040-X
- Healing Your Heart with Archangel Chamuel   1-84409-041-8

All available from your local bookshop,
or directly from www.findhornpress.com

For up-to-date information on Elisabeth Constantine's work and schedule,
please visit www.light-meditations.com

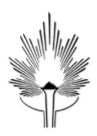

For further information about the Findhorn Foundation and the Findhorn Community,
please contact:

Findhorn Foundation
The Visitors Centre
The Park, Findhorn IV36 3TZ, Scotland, UK
tel 01309 690311
enquiries@findhorn.org
www.findhorn.org

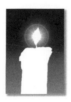

for a complete Findhorn Press catalogue, please contact:

Findhorn Press
305a The Park, Findhorn
Forres IV36 3TE
Scotland, UK
tel 01309 690582
fax 01309 690036
info@findhornpress.com
www.findhornpress.com